Urinary Continence and Sexual Function After Robotic Radical Prostatectomy

Sanjay Razdan

Editor

Urinary Continence and Sexual Function After Robotic Radical Prostatectomy

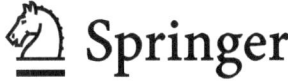 Springer

Editor
Sanjay Razdan, MD, MCh
International Robotic Prostatectomy Institute
Urology Center of Excellence at Jackson
    South Hospital
Miami, FL, USA

Videos to this book can be accessed at http://link.springer.com/book/10.1007/978-3-319-39448-0

ISBN 978-3-319-39446-6   ISBN 978-3-319-39448-0   (eBook)
DOI 10.1007/978-3-319-39448-0

Library of Congress Control Number: 2016951639

Printed on acid-free paper

This Springer imprint is published by Springer Nature
The registered company is Springer International Publishing AG Switzerland

Preface

The field of robotic prostatectomy is a rapidly evolving one. Newer techniques are allowing for shorter hospital times, faster recovery, and improved continence and erectile function. The speed at which surgical techniques and pre- and postoperative preparation are advancing is what prompted me to write this book. In it, I cover both the basics of robotic prostatectomy and the methods used by internationally recognized leaders in the field to maximize continence and erectile function. For truly, we are in a stage of medical and surgical practice in which curing the cancer is easy. Now we shift our focus to minimizing collateral damage.

The next frontier of robotic prostate surgery most definitely is not just curing the cancer, but also improving outcomes—with preserved continence and erectile function being at the top of a patient's priority list. With that in mind, this novel book is the first treatise in the world dedicated solely to the early return of continence and erectile function after robotic prostate surgery. The text is divided into 9 chapters, starting from the basic understanding of the anatomy and physiology of continence and potency and gradually evolving into the newer techniques to improve and hasten recovery of continence and erectile function.

What I found particularly useful while I was honing my personal surgical technique was watching videos of my surgeries and the videos of other experienced surgeons. In this manner, I was able to see what worked and what did not, and then tweak my procedure.

This is why we have included a series of videos as a companion to this book to help guide your study. Many chapters include references to videos that present the key points of each chapter. It is our hope that the reader finds these videos helpful.

At the end of the day, the most important thing to remember in robotic prostate surgery is to keep practicing. Even if a surgeon is not sitting at the console, maneuvering the joystick, and pressing the foot pedal, he or she can continue to watch videos, study the literature, and be open to dialogue with colleagues in the field of urologic oncology and perhaps even in other fields. In fact, it was a chance discussion with a neurosurgeon that prompted me to pioneer the use of human amniotic membrane in preserving nerve function during robotic prostatectomy, as will be discussed in Chap. 9. In due time, the novice will become an expert and will be devising their own techniques to better improve outcomes, as the surgeons who have contributed to this book have done.

I would like to thank my colleagues for generously contributing chapters to this book. Each and every chapter has been very well written by colleagues who I hold in high esteem for their outstanding contribution to robotic prostate surgery. It was truly a collaborative effort. I would also like to thank my family for their tireless support, particularly my daughter Shirin, for taking time out of her busy medical school schedule to help me and my fellows organize our vast database of patients who have undergone robotic prostatectomies.

We the authors hope you enjoy this textbook. We took pains to make it relevant to today's practice and understandable to surgeons at all levels of the learning curve. The videos that accompany the book should not be ignored, for they may even better show concepts explained in the chapters.

Our best wishes are with you.

Miami, FL, USA   Sanjay Razdan, MD, MCh

Contents

Contributors

Thomas E. Ahlering, MD Department of Urology, Irvine Medical Center, University of California, Irvine, Orange, CA, USA

Simone Albisinni, MD Department of Urology, Institut Jules Bordet, Brussels, Belgium

Fouad Aoun, MD, MSc Department of Urology, Institut Jules Bordet, Brussels, Belgium

Saint Joseph University, Hotel Dieu de France, Beirut, Lebanon

Nizar Boudiab, MD International Robotic Prostatectomy Institute, Urology Center of Excellence at Jackson South Hospital, Miami, FL, USA

Deepansh Dalela, MD VUI Center for Outcomes Research, Analytics and Evaluation, Vattikuti Urology Institute, Henry Ford Health System, Detroit, MI, USA

H.S. Dev University of Cambridge, Cambridge, UK

Louis Eichel, MD Division of Urology, Rochester General Hospital, Rochester, NY, USA

Center for Urology, Rochester, NY, USA

Hariharan Ganapathi Global Robotics Institute, Florida Hospital-Celebration Health, Celebration, FL, USA

Usama Khater, MD International Robotic Prostatectomy Institute, Urology Center of Excellence at Jackson South Hospital, Miami, FL, USA

Rose Khavari, MD Urology, Weill Cornell Medical College, Houston, TX, USA

Weil R. Lai, MD Department of Urology, Tulane University School of Medicine, New Orleans, LA, USA

Ksenija Limani, MD Department of Urology, Institut Jules Bordet, Brussels, Belgium

Mani Menon, MD VUI Center for Outcomes Research, Analytics and Evaluation, Vattikuti Urology Institute, Henry Ford Health System, Detroit, MI, USA

Brian J. Miles, MD Urology, Weill Cornell Medical College, Houston, TX, USA

Vladimir Mouraviev Global Robotics Institute, Florida Hospital-Celebration Health, Celebration, FL, USA

Gabriel Ogaya-Pinies Global Robotics Institute, Florida Hospital-Celebration Health, Celebration, FL, USA

Vipul Patel Global Robotics Institute, Florida Hospital-Celebration Health, Celebration, FL, USA

Sanjay Razdan, MD, MCh International Robotic Prostatectomy Institute, Urology Center of Excellence at Jackson South Hospital, Miami, FL, USA

Shirin Razdan, BS University of Miami Miller School of Medicine, Miami, FL, USA

Douglas Skarecky, BS Department of Urology, Irvine Medical Center, University of California, Irvine, Orange, CA, USA

P. Sooriakumaran, BMBS (Hons), MRCS, PhD, FRCSUrol, FEBU Nuffield Department of Surgical Sciences, University of Oxford, Oxford, Oxfordshire, UK

Raju Thomas, MD, FACS, MHA Department of Urology, Tulane University School of Medicine, New Orleans, LA, USA

Roland van Velthoven, MD, PhD Department of Urology, Institut Jules Bordet, Brussels, Belgium

P. Wiklund, MD, PhD Karolinska Institute, Stockholm, Sweden

Chapter 1
Anatomic Foundations and Physiology of Erectile Function and Urinary Continence

Deepansh Dalela and Mani Menon

The widespread use of PSA screening since the 1990s and the consequent downward stage migration of incident prostate cancer (PCa) in the United States has led to an increasing number of younger patients undergoing radical prostatectomy for clinically localized PCa. While this has led to higher disease specific and overall survival, it has also highlighted the critical role of functional outcomes (i.e., urinary continence and erectile function) in affecting the health-related quality of life for the PCa survivor. It is in this context that robot-assisted laparoscopic surgery offers tremendous opportunities, with its magnified, 3-dimensional view, more degree of freedom of movements, and the ability to carry out precise tissue dissections. The ability to translate these technological advancements into superior functional outcomes is, however, firmly predicated on a clear understanding of the underlying principles of anatomical and physiological interactions responsible for maintaining urinary continence and erectile function. This chapter is intended to discuss the evolution of current understanding of these aspects.

Anatomical Principles for Preservation of Erectile Function

Erectile bodies (corpora cavernosa) of the penis derive arterial blood from cavernosal artery and the dorsal penile artery (circumflex branches), both branches of the common penile artery (which itself is derived from the internal pudendal artery). Venous blood from the endothelial-lined sinusoids of the cavernosal bodies drains into the subtunical capillary plexus, emissary veins from which ultimately join the deep dorsal vein. The autonomic nerves supplying the cavernosal bodies are derived

D. Dalela, M.D. (✉) • M. Menon, M.D.
VUI Center for Outcomes Research, Analytics and Evaluation, Vattikuti Urology Institute, Henry Ford Health System, 2799 West Grand Boulevard, K-9, Detroit, MI 48202, USA
e-mail: ddalela1@hfhs.org

© Springer International Publishing Switzerland 2016
S. Razdan (ed.), *Urinary Continence and Sexual Function After Robotic Radical Prostatectomy*, DOI 10.1007/978-3-319-39448-0_1

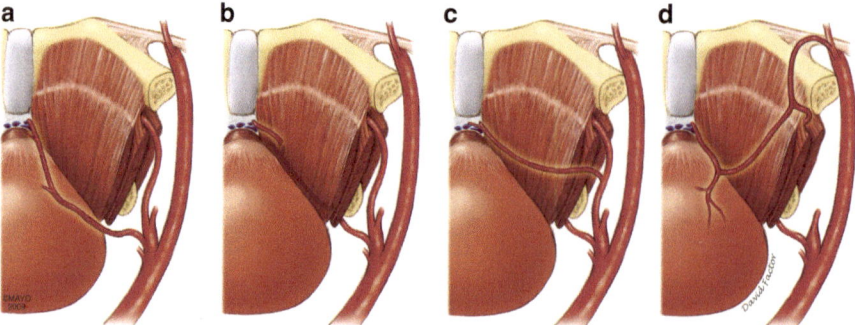

Fig. 1.1 Aberrant and accessory pudendal arteries: (**a**) aberrant lateral supralevator pudendal artery branching from internal iliac artery; (**b**) accessory apical pudendal artery branching from infralevator pudendal artery; (**c**) accessory lateral pudendal artery branching from obturator artery; (**d**) accessory pudendal artery branching from external iliac artery with aberrant obturator and infravesical branches. (From Walz J, Burnett AL, Costello AJ, Eastham JA, Graefen M, Guillonneau B, et al. A critical analysis of the current knowledge of surgical anatomy related to optimization of cancer control and preservation of continence and erection in candidates for radical prostatectomy. Eur Urol. 2010 Feb;57(2):179–92) (Reproduced, with permission, from Elsevier)

from the pelvic plexus (or the inferior hypogastric plexus), which is responsible for erection, ejaculation, and urinary continence. The parasympathetic preganglionic fibers ('nervi erigentes') to the plexus originate from the intermediolateral horns of the S2–S4 spinal cord segments and are responsible for vasodilation and increased blood flow during erection, while the sympathetic fibers from the thoracolumbar outflow (T11–L2) reach the pelvic plexus through the hypogastric nerve and are mainly responsible for ejaculation. The pelvic plexus is a 4–5 cm long rectangular plate, located in the sagittal plane in the groove between the rectum and the bladder, with its midpoint corresponding to the tips of the seminal vesicles and the most caudal part giving rise to the cavernous nerves regulating erectile function. Besides the corpora cavernosa, the pelvic plexus provides autonomic innervation to the urinary bladder, ureter, seminal vesicles, prostate, rectum, and external urethral sphincter.

Given that the key elements of erection involve increased blood flow to the penis following neural stimulation, disturbance to the vascular or neural elements of this phenomenon is likely to cause impotence or erectile dysfunction. Although the major arterial supply of the penis is derived from the internal pudendal artery, accessory or aberrant pudendal arteries (present in 4–75 % of men) may originate from the internal, external iliac, or obturator arteries and be the sole arterial blood supply to the corpora cavernosa (Fig. 1.1). Because these arteries course along the lower part of the bladder and the anterolateral surface of the prostate, they are at risk of injury during RP resulting in 'vasculogenic' erectile dysfunction [1, 2]. On the other hand, injury to the autonomic nerves supplying the cavernosal bodies, either by direct transection, cautery, or traction, can result in 'neurogenic' erectile dysfunction. Unfortunately, until the 1980s, the detailed topographical relationship of nerve fibers from the pelvic plexus to their cavernosal bodies was not well understood, which contributed to the high rates of postoperative impotence. Indeed, initial descriptions of radical perineal prostatectomy by Young, Higbee, and Colston were marked by almost universal loss of sexual function after surgery.

Presence of Anatomically Distinct Neurovascular Bundles

The first reference to the existence of erectogenic neural bundles (supplying the cavernosal bodies) was made by the German anatomist Johannes Muller in 1836 through vivid illustrations in his text book 'The organic nerves of male sexual organ of human and mammals' [3]. Not only did he differentiate between autonomic and somatic innervation of the pelvic and genital organs, but also stated that "organic cavernosal nerves do not follow the course of the vessels into the phallus but have a much shorter course." Although this was followed by neurophysiological studies of the pelvic plexus in the later part of the nineteenth century, its implications in radical prostatectomy were revived by Alex Finkle in 1960 [4] when he emphasized that sharp lateral transection through both layers of Denonvilliers' fascia at or proximal to distal ends of seminal vesicles during radical perineal prostatectomy almost inevitably damages parasympathetic fibers. However, it was the seminal work by Walsh and colleagues in the 1980s [5–7] that ushered in the era of nerve sparing radical prostatectomy.

Based on a series of dissections performed on the male fetus and newborn, Walsh and Donker [6] noted that the branches of inferior vesical artery and vein (which divide to supply the bladder and the prostate) perforate the pelvic plexus. They also traced the course of cavernosal nerves, traveling posterolateral to the prostate on the surface of rectum and lateral to the prostatic capsular vessels (hence constituting the term 'neurovascular bundle' [NVB]), and lying within and adjacent to the membranous urethra at the level of the apex. While noting the absence of vasculogenic causes in postprostatectomy erectile dysfunction, they suggested that injury to the pelvic plexus at two distinct sites to be the main contributory factor: one, during ligation and division of the lateral pedicle of prostate and bladder in its mid-portion (which may injure nerves innervating prostate, urethra, and corpora cavernosa), and two, during apical dissection and transection of urethra and surrounding tissues (which may specifically damage the cavernosal nerves). The NVB was observed to be located in a triangular space between the two layers of the lateral pelvic fascia (levator fascia [lateral layer] and prostatic fascia [medial layer]) and the anterior layer of the Denonvilliers' fascia forming the posterior boundary, and during a nerve-sparing procedure, the prostatic fascia was excised. While the plane of dissection for a radical perineal prostatectomy was maintained below the levator fascia, a retropubic approach entailed approaching the prostate from outside the lateral pelvic fascia, incising the fascia posterolaterally but sufficiently anterior to the NVB, followed by the division of the lateral pedicle close to the prostate to prevent injury to the NVB [7].

Expansion of the Neuroanatomical Principles

Aided by the magnification and 3-dimensional vision afforded by the robot, Menon's group, that had already established the world's first robotic surgery training program in 2001 [8], undertook a detailed cadaveric study of the periprostatic neuroanatomy to provide a roadmap for nerve preservation for the surgeon performing laparoscopic or radical prostatectomy [9]. They noted the existence of the multilayered periprostatic fascia, the most prominent of which were the prostatic fascia medially and the lateral pelvic fascia laterally. While the main NVB was enclosed between these two layers and the Denonvilliers' fascia posterolateral to the prostate, multiple smaller nerves ramify within the layers of periprostatic fascia all along the surface of the prostate (Fig. 1.2). Additionally, unlike Walsh, who suggested a retrograde approach to nerve dissection (beginning from the apex and moving upward), Menon's group supported an antegrade dissection of NVB, since the triangular space containing the NVB was noted to be broader at the base than the apex (Fig. 1.3). Other investigators too described significant variations in the classical NVB description of periprostatic nerve fibers, and some of the relevant findings are summarized in Table 1.1.

Toward the apical region of the prostate, the NVB lies in close relation to the urethral sphincter and prostate apex [6]. While the number of fibers at apex is less than that at base, they surround the sphicteric urethra up to the 2 o'clock and 10 o' clock positions [18] (Fig. 1.6), though mainly concentrated at 4–5 o' clock and 7–8 o' clock positions [19]. The ventral aspect of the apex and the urethra (which is covered by the rhabdosphincteric fascia), and the dorsal median raphe of the rhabdosphincter, are free of nerve fibers, providing an important avascular plane of dissection [18].

With increasing recognition of cavernous nerves spread over the anterolateral surface of the prostate (extending from 2 o' clock to the 10 o' clock position, instead of being confined to the posterolateral 5 and 7 o' clock location), and better understanding of periprostatic neural anatomy as the nerves course from the base toward the apex, some investigators suggested incising the pelvic fascia much more anteriorly than the classic Walsh technique [9, 14, 15, 19]. Costello et al. [20] had also shown by immunohistochemical staining of periprostatic nerve fibers that while the relative proportion of parasympathetic, sympathetic, and somatic nerve fibers on the anterior and anterolateral surface of the prostate was 14.3, 55.7, and 30 % respectively, this changed to 23.1, 52.3, and 18.6 % at the level of the prostatic apex. It was thus possible that some of the parasympathetic fibers 'swung' anteriorly along their cephalo-caudal course over the surface of the prostate. Montorsi et al. [19] reported continence (0–1 urinary pad per day) and potency (erectile function domain score of the International Index of Erectile Function [IIEF] ≥26) rates of 90 and 52 %, respectively, with the high anterior release (HAR) technique (incising the levator and prostatic fasciae high anteriorly at 1 and 11 o' clock positions), with lower positive surgical margins (PSM; 14.3 %) than historical cohorts. Around the same time, building upon the detailed neuroanatomical understanding afforded by the robotic platform, Menon et al. [9, 21, 22] were the first to describe their results with preservation of nerves in the lateral periprostatic fascia, eponymously titled "the Veil

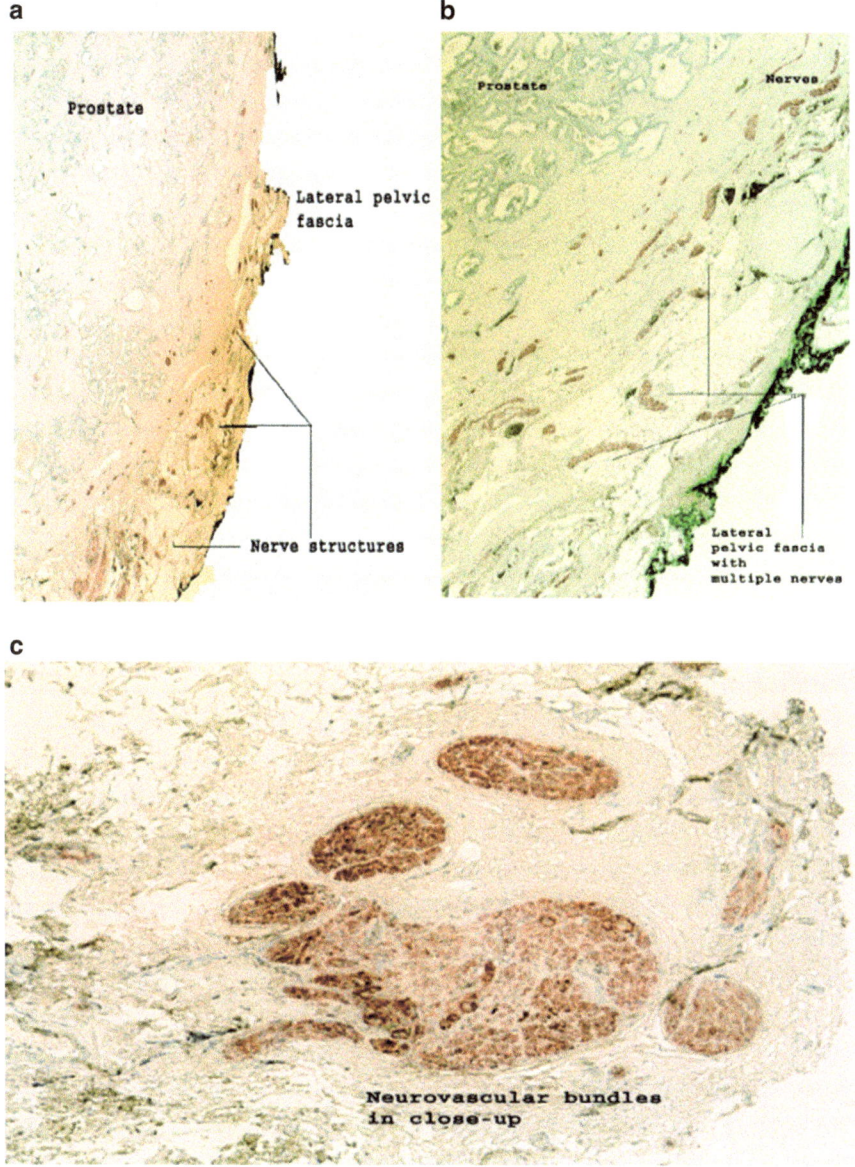

Fig. 1.2 Microscopic images of the nerves in the lateral pelvic fascia (brown structures) (note the small nerves posterior and anterolateral to the prostate): (**a**) low magnification; (**b**) medium magnification; (**c**) high magnification. (Reproduced, with permission, from Elsevier [Tewari et al.])

of Aphrodite" technique: dissecting in a plane between the prostatic capsule and the periprostatic fascia, they noted 96 % of pre-operatively potent men had erections sufficient for intercourse 12 months after surgery. Likewise, Walsh [23] and later Myers [24] reported comparable potency rates of 67–70 % (defined as return to baseline

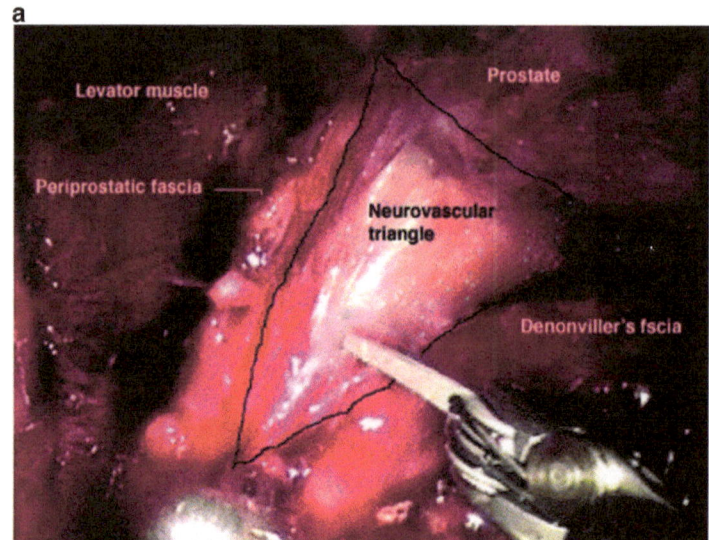

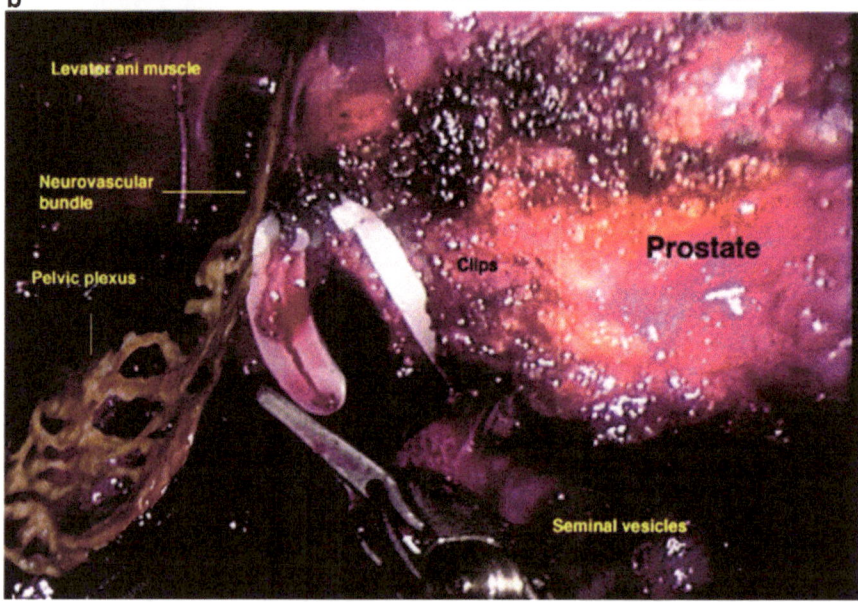

Fig. 1.3 Computer enhanced intraoperative relationship between the lateral pelvic fascia, Denonvillier's fascia, and prostate and neurovascular bundles: (**a**) triangle of lateral pelvic fascia, prostate, and Denonvillier's sheet and their relationship with nerves; (**b**) relationship between pelvic plexus and neurovascular bundles to the left prostatic pedicle. (Reproduced, with permission, from Elsevier [Tewari et al.])

Sexual Health Inventory for Men [SHIM] score ≥22) at 1 year with the HAR of levator fascia, without compromising the surgical margins of the resected tumor (in contrast to Menon et al. [22], the plane of dissection adopted by the aforementioned authors was between the prostatic and levator ani fascia).

Table 1.1 Key variations described in the distribution of neurovascular bundles and periprostatic nerve fibers

Author/investigator	Key findings
Costello et al. [10]	Suggested three functional components of the NVBs in distinct fascial compartments: the posterior/posterolateral component that runs within the Denonvilliers' and pararectal fascia and innervates the rectum, a second lateral component innervating the levator ani, and a third anterior component comprising the cavernosal nerves and prostatic neurovascular supply (the component that was originally described by Walsh)
Kourambas et al. [11]	Nerves scattered throughout the Denonvilliers' fascia, including medially toward the midline
Kiyoshima et al. [12]	Varying amounts of adipose tissue interposed between prostatic capsule and prostatic fascia in nearly half the cases (48 %): a lattice of nerve fibers was distributed over the anterolateral surface of the prostate, deep to the prostatic fascia
Takenaka et al. [13]	Periprostatic nerves distributed on the lateral surface of the prostate, showing a spray-like arrangement rather than distinct NVB formation
Lunacek et al. [14]	NVB dispersed over the convex surface of the prostate (like a curtain) during embryonic growth: incision of periprostatic fascia and dissection of NVB performed anteriorly (curtain dissection) (Fig. 1.4)
Eichelberg et al. [15]	Only 46–66 % of all nerves found in posterolateral location, while 21–29 % located over the anterolateral surface of the prostate
Tewari et al. [16]	Trizonal, "hammock" like distribution of periprostatic nerves: the proximal neurovascular plate (another name for the pelvic plexus), the predominant neurovascular bundle and the accessory neural pathways (observed anterolaterally between prostatic and lateral pelvic fascia, in several planes between the layers of periprostatic fascia, and posteriorly within the layers of Denonvilliers' fascia) (Fig. 1.5)
Ganzer et al. [17]	The percentage of total nerve surface area was highest dorsolaterally (84.1, 75.1, and 74.5 % at the base, middle, and apex, respectively), but this finding was variable. Up to 39.9 % of nerve surface area was found ventrolaterally and up to 45.5 % in the dorsal position

Alsaid et al. [25], in an elegantly performed study in human male fetuses and adult cadavers, performed serial transverse sections of the pelvis (Fig. 1.7) and stained them with S-100 to localize the path of the periprostatic nerves as they enter the penile hilum. These serial sections were then reconstructed into computer-aided 3-dimensional images, and the authors noted that beyond the prostatic apex, the NVB divided into cavernosal nerves (CN) and corpora spongiosa nerves (CSN) (Fig. 1.8). In contradistinction to all the preceding studies, the authors observed that the CNs were continuation of the anterior and anterolateral periprostatic nerve fibers, and the CSN were derived mostly from the posterolateral NVBs. However, more than 50 % of nerve fibers located on the anterior surface of the prostate were found to be sympathetic in Costello's study [20] and may plausibly be thought to innervate the prostatic stroma, nearby vascular structures and the external urethral sphincter, rather than supply the cavernosal bodies. As such, the rationale for the HAR or the Veil technique might be less neuropraxic and thermal injury (since the

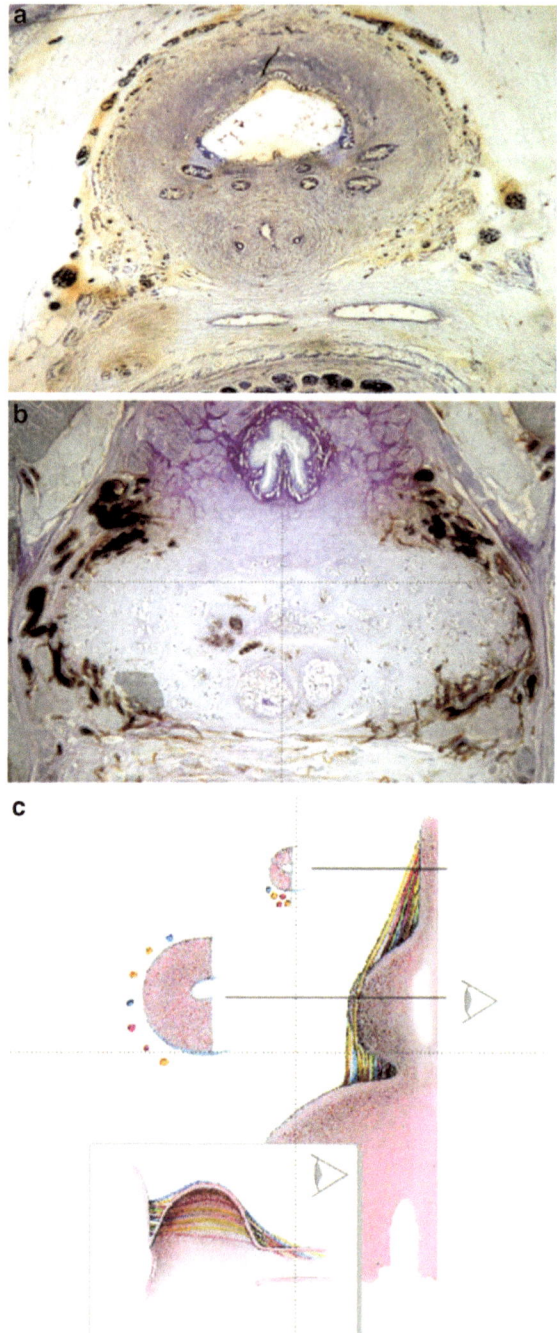

Fig. 1.4 Change of course of the CNs during development of the prostate. The vessels are filled with darkly stained erythrocytes, the CNs are situated between and around the periprostatic vessels. (**a**) Fetal specimen, transverse section, 13 weeks. Before development of the prostate the CNs

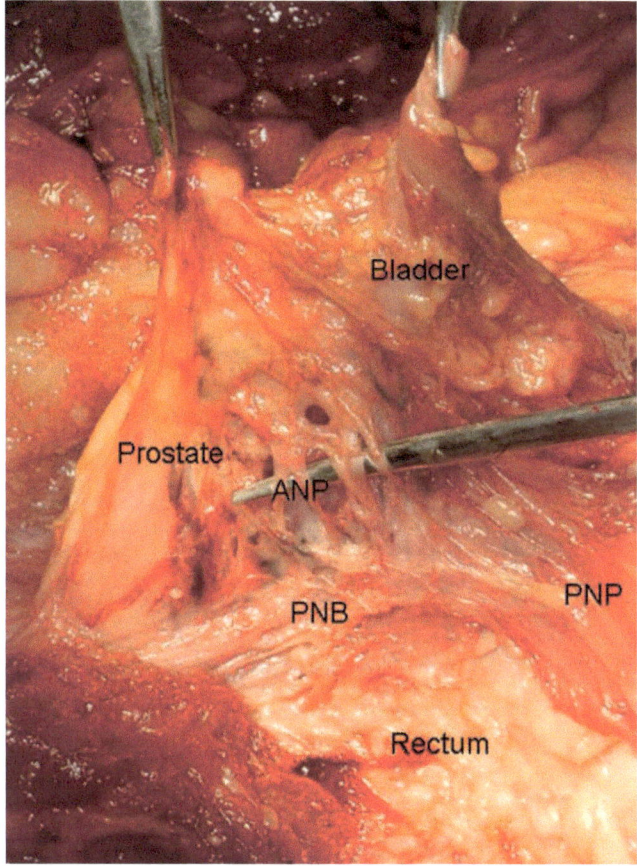

Fig. 1.5 Lateral view of PNP, PNB, and ANP. Fresh cadaver dissection showing that the neural pathway from the PNP is a spray-like distribution. The prostate and bladder are lifted up by the forceps. (Reproduced, with permission, from Wiley [Tewari et al.])

Fig. 1.4 (continued) (marked with *asterisks*) are situated lateral and dorsal to the future prostatic (PU) and membranous urethra, as well as the rhabdosphincter (RS). All around the urethra darkly stained blood vessels can be seen. (**b**) Fetal specimen, transverse section, 22 weeks. Because of the growth of the prostate (P) the CNs (marked with *asterisks*) and the blood vessels (with darkly stained erythrocytes) running in the NVB are increasingly dispersed along the convex surface of the prostate. Therefore, they now assume a concave 'curtain' shape. *U* urethra, *RS* rhabdosphincter. (**c**) Drawing of the concave 'curtain' shape of the NVB after development and growth of the prostate. The two cross-sections show the course of the NVB along the surface of the prostate and along the dorsolateral aspect of the membranous urethra. The *red arrow* marks the anterior site of incision of the lateral pelvic fascia during the new 'curtain dissection' of the NVB. The *blue arrow* shows the far more dorsally situated standard site of dissection of the NVB. The *asterisks* mark the CNs that are situated along the surface of the prostate and dorsolateral to the membranous urethra. In the smaller drawing the NVB situated in the lateral pelvic fascia is shown after removing the prostate. (Reproduced, with permission, from Wiley [Lunacek et al.])

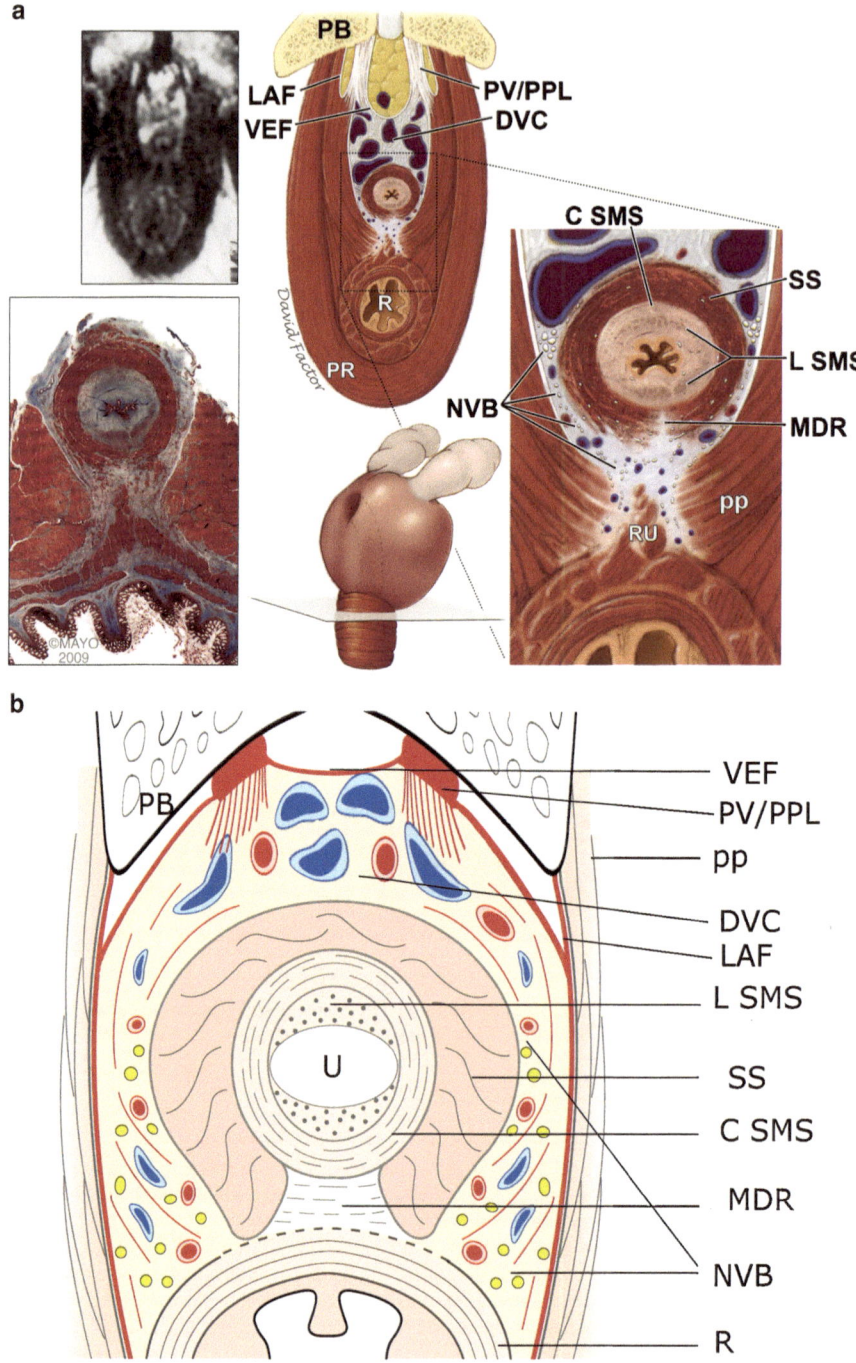

Fig. 1.6 Axial section of sphincteric urethra: (**a**) anatomic; (**b**) schematic. *DVC* dorsal vascular complex, *LAF* levator ani fascia, *MDR* median dorsal raphe, *NVB* neurovascular bundle, *PB* pubic bone, *PV/PPL* pubovesical/puboprostatic ligament, *pp* puboperinealis muscle, *PR* puborectalis muscle, *R* rectum, *RU* rectourethralis muscle, *SS* striated sphincter (rhabdosphincter); *C SMS* circular smooth muscle sphincter (lissosphincter), *L SMS* longitudinal smooth muscle sphincter (lissosphincter), *U* urethra, *VEF* visceral endopelvic fascia. (From Walz J, Burnett AL, Costello AJ, Eastham JA, Graefen M, Guillonneau B, et al. A critical analysis of the current knowledge of surgical anatomy related to optimization of cancer control and preservation of continence and erection in candidates for radical prostatectomy. Eur Urol. 2010 Feb;57(2):179–92) (Reproduced, with permission, from Elsevier)

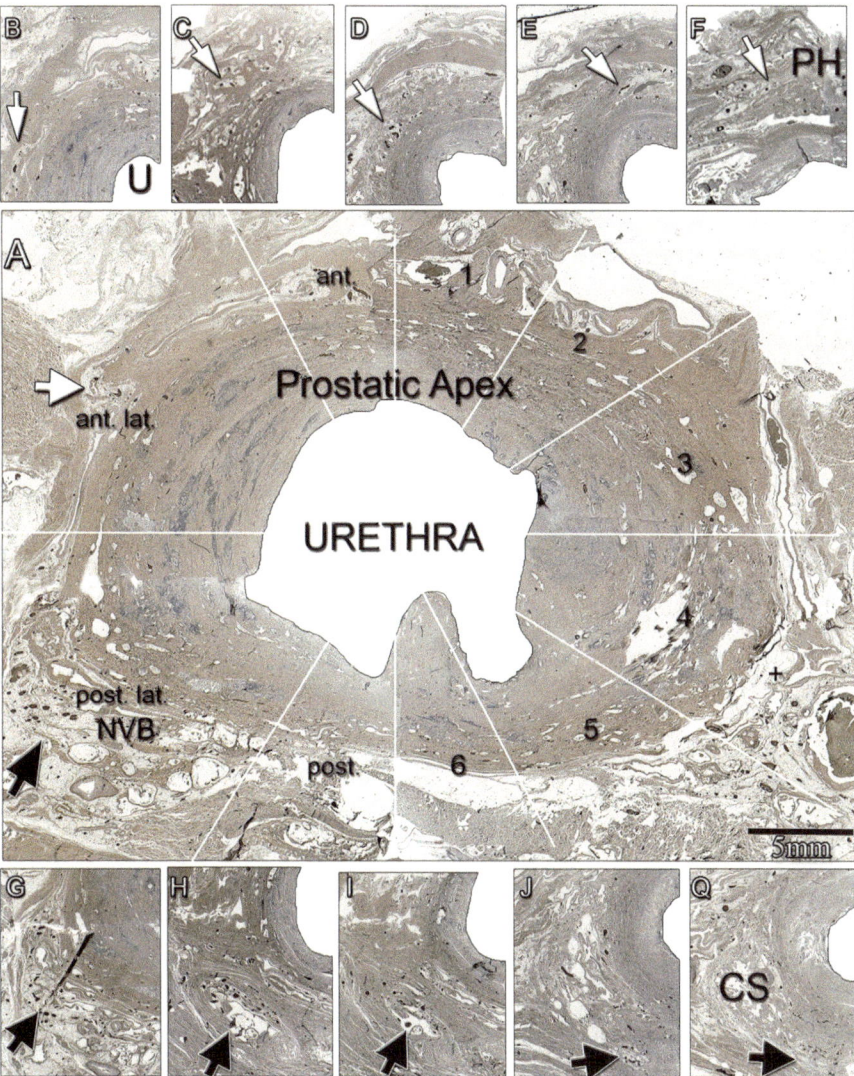

Fig. 1.7 (**a**) Histologic transverse section of 72-year-old adult cadaver at the level of the prostate apex, immunolabeled with anti-S100 antibody and scanned at an optical resolution of 3200 dpi. On the *right*, sector division in a clockwise direction (1–6 o'clock); on the *left*, the corresponding anterior (ant.), anterolateral (ant. lat.), posterolateral (post. lat.), and posterior (post.) regions, classical position of the neurovascular bundle (NVBs) in the posterolateral regions (*back arrow*), location of fibers in the anterolateral regions (*white arrow*). (**b–q**) Serial histologic transverse sections (4 mm apart) between the membranous urethra (U) and corpus spongiosum levels, with some of the anterolateral nerve fibres (B–F, white arrows) travelling toward the penile hilum (PH) and the corpora cavernosa. The posterolateral nerve fibers (G–Q, black arrows) form the distal course of the NVBs and reach the corpus spongiosum (CS). (From Alsaid B, Bessede T, Diallo D, Moszkowicz D, Karam I, Benoit G, et al. Division of autonomic nerves within the neurovascular bundles distally into corpora cavernosa and corpus spongiosum components: immunohistochemical confirmation with three-dimensional reconstruction. Eur Urol. 2011 Jun;59(6):902–9) (Reproduced, with permission, from Elsevier)

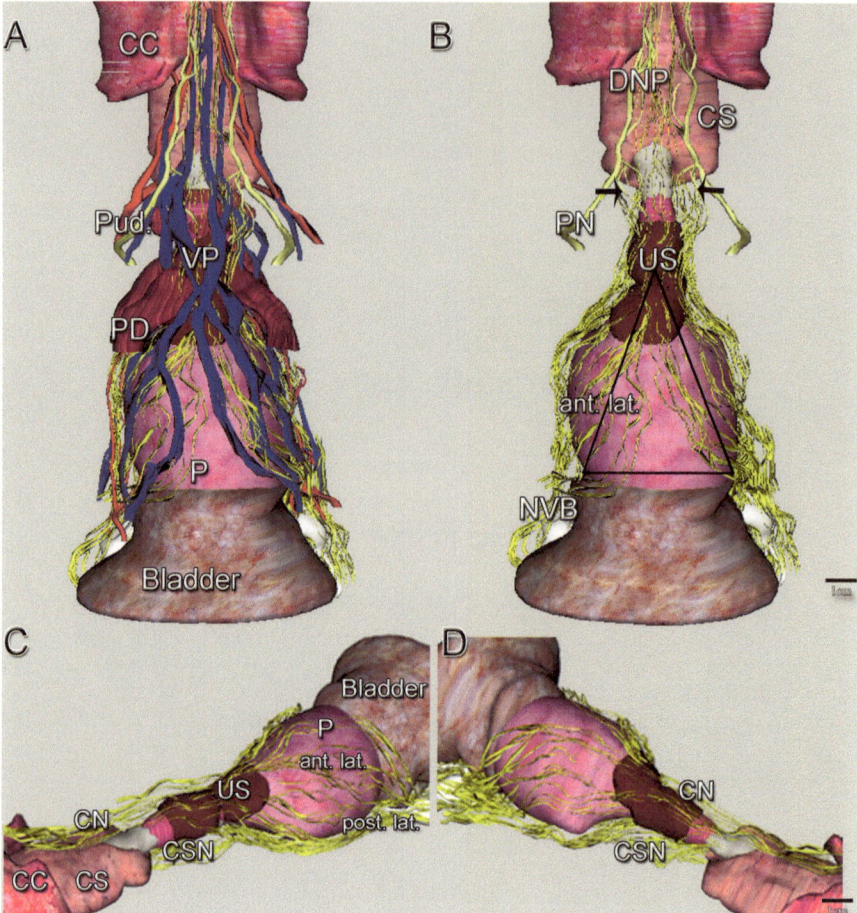

Fig. 1.8 Three-dimensional computer-assisted anatomic dissection from transverse immunola-beled histologic sections of a cadaver of a 74-years-old man. (**b**) Superior view of intrapelvic organs showing supralevator and the distal part of infralevator neurovascular pathways; (**b**) same view without the pelvic diaphragm (PD), the pudendal vessels (Pud.), and the venous plexus (VP). The pudendal nerve (PN) innervates the urethral sphincter (US) before becoming the dorsal nerve of the penis (DNP). Branches from the PN intermingle with the cavernous nerves, forming a caverno-pudendal distal communication (*black arrows*). The neurovascular bundles (NVBs) are located in their classical position, posterolateral to the base of the prostate (P). Nerve fibers are also found in anterior and anterolateral (ant. lat.) positions, following the lateral edges of a triangle (*black triangle*) with its tip at the apex of the prostate. (**c**) Right anterolateral and (**d**) left anterolat-eral views of the supralevator nerve pathways. The NVBs contain two divisions: the cavernous nerves (CNs), forming a continuation of the anterolateral fibers extending toward the corpora cav-ernosa (CC) and the penile hilum, and the corpus spongiosum nerves (CSNs), which represent the distal course of the posterolateral (post. lat.) NVBs reaching the corpus spongiosum bulb (CS). (From Alsaid B, Bessede T, Diallo D, Moszkowicz D, Karam I, Benoit G, et al. Division of auto-nomic nerves within the neurovascular bundles distally into corpora cavernosa and corpus spon-giosum components: immunohistochemical confirmation with three-dimensional reconstruction. Eur Urol. 2011 Jun;59(6):902–9) (Reproduced, with permission, from Elsevier)

incision is made far away from the posterolateral NVB) and better vascular control, rather than preservation of functional ventrally placed nerves perse. Another possibility is that preservation of prostatic fascia maintains additional vascular supply to the cavernosal bodies or the cavernosal nerves [22]. Regardless, the HAR and Veil techniques have conclusively shown that in the hands of an experienced surgeon and with appropriate patient selection, optimal potency outcomes may be achievable without compromising the oncologic efficacy of the operation.

Fascial Anatomy of the Prostate

Endopelvic Fascia

The pelvic organs are covered by the endopelvic fascia, which can either be parietal or visceral. The parietal aspect lines the inner surface of pelvic muscles and is continuous with fascia transversalis of the abdomen. The inner or the visceral layer covers the pelvic organs, including the prostate, bladder, and rectum and fuses with the anterior fibromuscular layer of the prostate at the upper ventral aspect of the gland [18]. The parietal and visceral layers are fused along the pelvic sidewall, and the fascial condensation is known as fascial tendinous arch of pelvis (FTAP) (Figs. 1.6 and 1.9), extending from the puboprostatic ligaments (PPL) to the ischial spine. Incision made lateral to the FTAP incises the levator ani fascia strips the muscle fibers of their fascial covering, while bringing levator ani fascia in direct approximation with the prostatic fascia (Fig. 1.10). Conversely, a medial incision on the visceral endopelvic fascia leaves the levator ani fascia intact on the muscle, while the prostate is covered only by the prostatic fascia [18].

Periprostatic Fascia

Traditionally referred to by a confusing array of similar sounding terms (such as the lateral pelvic fascia, periprostatic fascia, parapelvic fascia, or simply the prostatic fascia), the fascial covering immediately outside of the prostatic capsule is a complex, multilayered structure with fibrofatty elements. The anterior extension of the periprostatic fascia is represented by the visceral layer of endopelvic fascia covering the prostate between 10–11 o' clock and 1–2 o' clock positions, and merging with the anterior fibromuscular stroma in the midline. Laterally, it is represented by the layers of levator ani fascia and the prostatic fascia when the endopelvic fascia is incised lateral to the FTAP (Figs. 1.1 and 1.6). Finally, the posterior surface of the prostate and the seminal vesicles is covered by the posterior prostatic and the seminal vesicle fascia (popularly known as the Denonvilliers' fascia). The Denonvilliers' fascia extends superiorly from the base of rectovesical pouch to the apex of the prostate at the level of prostatourethral junction and merges caudally with the central perineal tendon. A cleavage plane may be developed between the Denonvilliers'

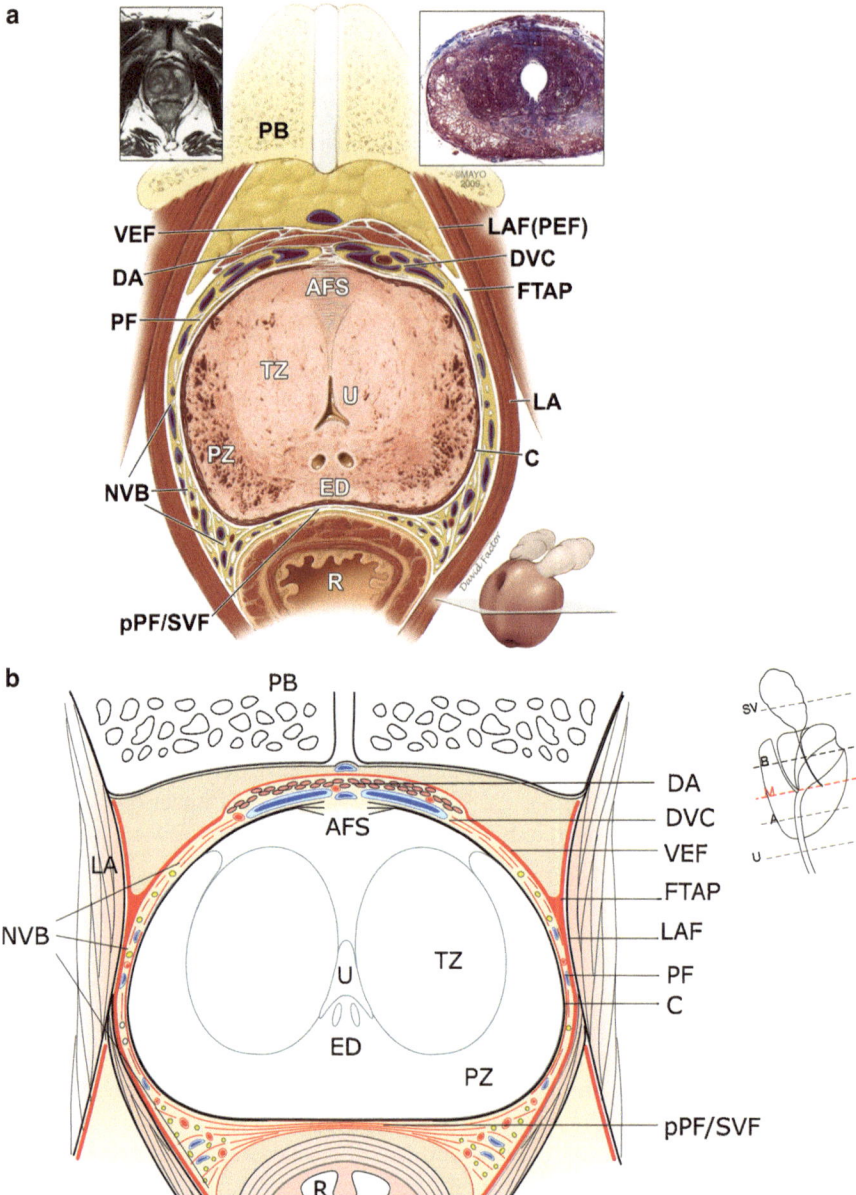

Fig. 1.9 Axial section of prostate and periprostatic fascias at midprostate: (**a**) anatomic; (**b**) schematic. *AFS* anterior fibromuscular stroma, *C* capsule of prostate, *DA* detrusor apron, *DVC* dorsal vascular complex, *ED* ejaculatory ducts, *FTAP* fascial tendinous arch of pelvis, *LA* levator ani muscle, *LAF* levator ani fascia, *NVB* neurovascular bundle, *PB* pubic bone, *PEF* parietal endopelvic fascia, *PF* prostatic fascia, *pPF/SVF* posterior prostatic fascia/seminal vesicles fascia (Denonvilliers' fascia); *PZ* peripheral zone, *R* rectum; *TZ* transition zone, *U* urethra; *VEF* visceral endopelvic fascia. (From Walz J, Burnett AL, Costello AJ, Eastham JA, Graefen M, Guillonneau B, et al. A critical analysis of the current knowledge of surgical anatomy related to optimization of cancer control and preservation of continence and erection in candidates for radical prostatectomy. Eur Urol. 2010 Feb;57(2):179–92) (Reproduced, with permission, from Elsevier)

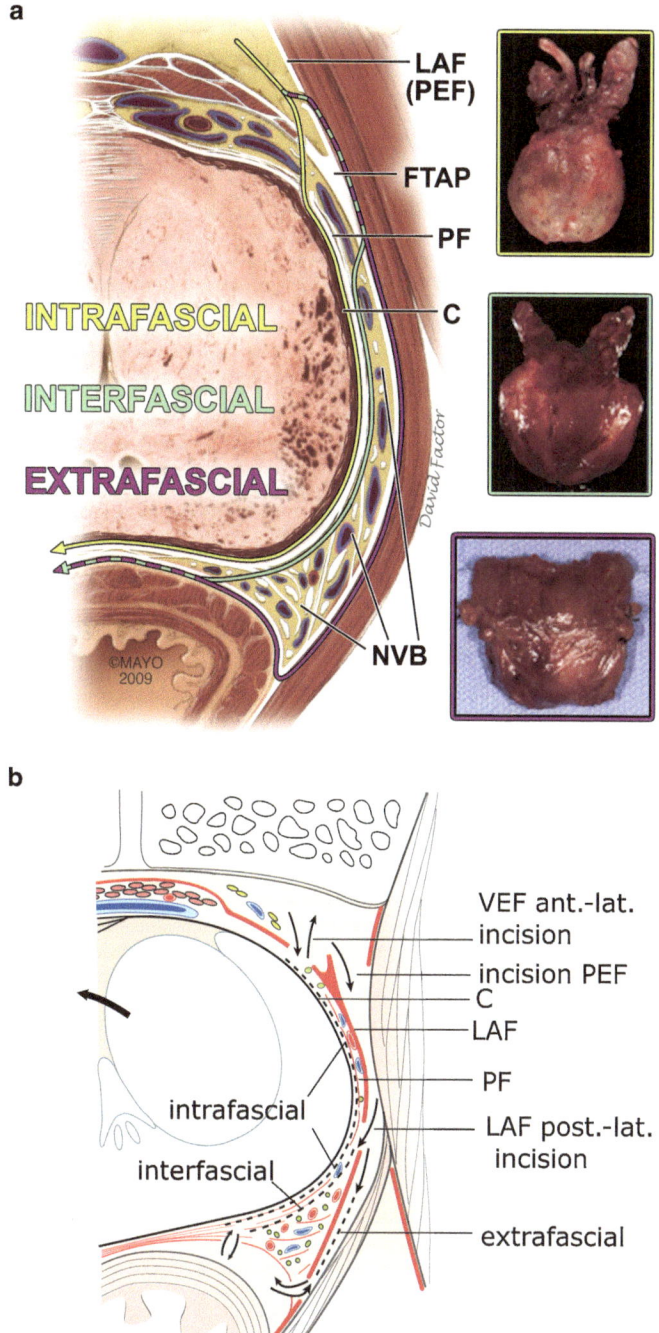

Fig. 1.10 Axial section of prostate and periprostatic fascias at midprostate with three different dissection planes demonstrated (intrafascial [*yellow line*], interfascial [*green line*], and extrafascial [*purple line*]): (**a**) anatomic, showing a high anterior release of interfascial dissection; (**b**) schematic (prostate rotated counterclockwise), showing the classical posterolateral release of interfascial dissection. *Insets* represent pure dissections with final specimens shown, although in practice, mixtures are commonplace. *C* capsule of prostate, *FTAP* fascial tendinous arch of pelvis, *LAF* levator ani fascia, *NVB* neurovascular bundle, *PEF* parietal endopelvic fascia, *PF* prostatic fascia, *VEF* visceral endopelvic fascia. (From Walz J, Burnett AL, Costello AJ, Eastham JA, Graefen M, Guillonneau B, et al. A critical analysis of the current knowledge of surgical anatomy related to optimization of cancer control and preservation of continence and erection in candidates for radical prostatectomy. Eur Urol. 2010 Feb;57(2):179–92) (Reproduced, with permission, from Elsevier)

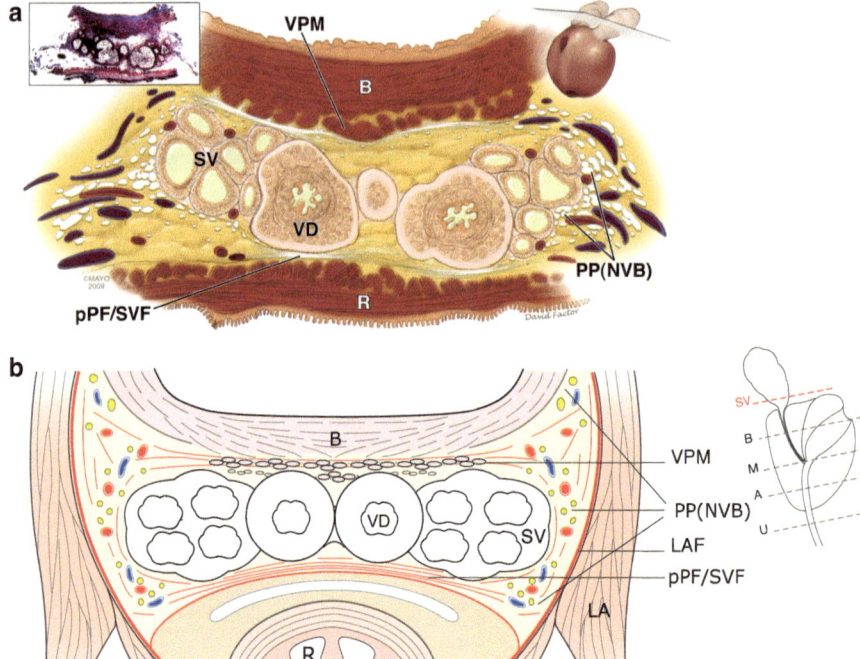

Fig. 1.11 Axial section through base of seminal vesicles to show proximity of distal pelvic plexus (neurovascular bundle [NVB]): (**a**) anatomic (**b**) schematic. *B* bladder; *PP* pelvic plexus, *pPF/SVF* posterior prostatic fascia/seminal vesicle fascia (Denonvilliers' fascia), *R* rectum, *SV* seminal vesicle, *VD* vas deferens, *VPM* vesicoprostatic muscle. (From Walz J, Burnett AL, Costello AJ, Eastham JA, Graefen M, Guillonneau B, et al. A critical analysis of the current knowledge of surgical anatomy related to optimization of cancer control and preservation of continence and erection in candidates for radical prostatectomy. Eur Urol. 2010 Feb;57(2):179–92) (Reproduced, with permission, from Elsevier)

fascia anteriorly and fascia propria of the rectum posteriorly during radical prostatectomy, owing to the possible distinct embryological origin of the latter by fusion of the two peritoneal layers of pouch of Douglas [26]. The Denonvilliers' fascia represents a musculofascial plate, consisting of collagenous, elastic, and smooth muscle fibers intermixed into a single-layered membrane. While the traditional location of the NVB has been described in the triangular space bounded laterally by the levator ani fascia, medially by the prostatic fascia and posteriorly by the Denonvilliers' fascia (Fig. 1.11), Kourambas et al. [11] suggested the existence of an "H" shaped structure: the upper limbs formed by right and left lateral periprostatic fasciae, lower limbs by right and left pararectal fasciae, and the horizontal limb formed by the Denonvilliers' fascia. The Denonvilliers' fascia then splits at its lateral border into anterior and posterior layers, enclosing the NVB in a triangular space bound laterally by the levator ani fascia [9, 10].

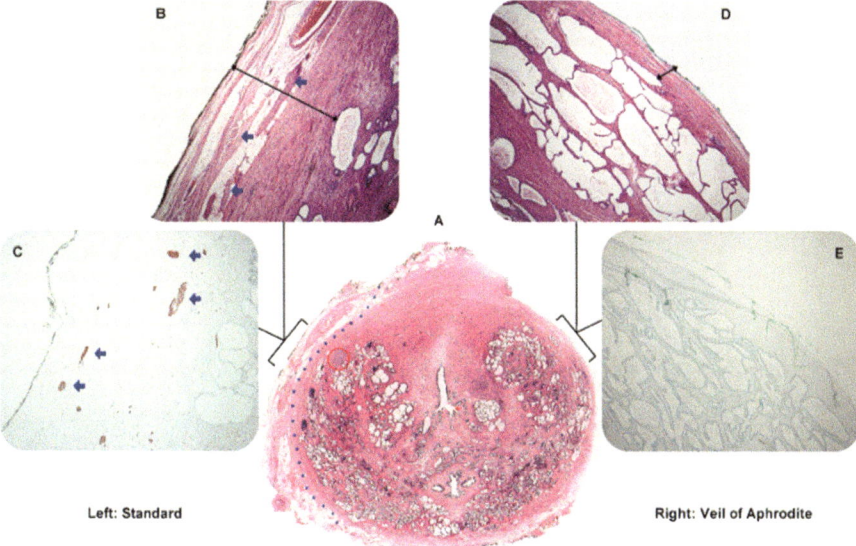

Fig. 1.12 Whole-mount section of prostate with standard technique (ST) on the *left* and Veil of Aphrodite technique (VT) on the *right*. (**a**) Entire whole-mount, hematoxylin and eosin (H&E). Note the tumor (*red circle*), presence of lateral prostatic fascia (LPF) on the *left*, and its absence on the *right*. For comparison, *blue dotted line* represents the plane of excision for VT, as has been done on the *right*. (**b**, H&E; **c**, S100; _40). Matching area of left AL zone. Note the LPF with nerve bundles (*blue arrows*). Margin clearance (*black arrow line*) is 1.6 mm. (**d**, H&E; **e**, S100; _40). Matching area of right AL zone. Note the absence of LPF and periprostatic nerve bundles. Margin clearance (*black arrow line*) is 0.3 mm. (From Savera AT, Kaul S, Badani K, Stark AT, Shah NL, Menon M. Robotic radical prostatectomy with the "Veil of Aphrodite" technique: histologic evidence of enhanced nerve sparing. Eur Urol. 2006 Jun;49(6):1065–73; discussion 73–4) (Reproduced, with permission, from Elsevier)

Intrafascial Dissection

Intrafascial dissection of the NVB entails dissection along the prostatic capsule, remaining deep to the prostatic fascia at the anterolateral and posterolateral aspects of prostate, as well as anterior to the Denonvilliers' fascia (Fig. 1.10). The intrafascial approach allows a whole thickness preservation of the lateral periprostatic fascia and therefore a complete preservation of the NVB because it remains covered by and lateral to the prostatic fascia. Identification of the prostatic fascia is obviously vital to the performance of this dissection, and the highly magnified, three-dimensional vision of the robotic system allows clear identification of the multiple layers of the prostatic fascia. Building upon the studies of Kiyoshima et al. [12], Menon [21, 22, 27] suggested nerve dissection in the plane between the prostatic fascia and the capsule (known as the "Veil of Aphrodite" sparing technique (Fig. 1.12)) beginning inferolaterally where the prostatic fascia reflects off the prostate, and

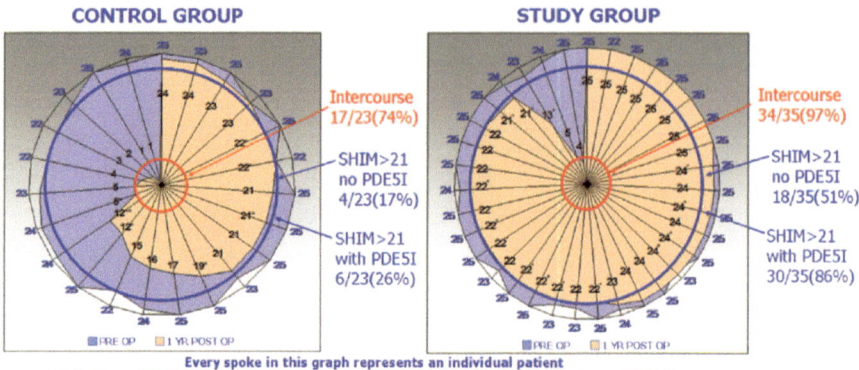

Fig. 1.13 Radar graph shows preoperative and postoperative SHIM scores in each patient (spokes) and ability of procedure to preserve sexual function. Extent of *blue* areas correlates with postoperative loss of potency. (From Menon M, Kaul S, Bhandari A, Shrivastava A, Tewari A, Hemal A. Potency following robotic radical prostatectomy: a questionnaire based analysis of outcomes after conventional nerve sparing and prostatic fascia sparing techniques. J Urol. 2005 Dec;174(6):2291–6, discussion 6) (Reproduced, with permission, from Elsevier)

proceeds in an antegrade fashion. The use of antegrade approach is facilitated by a 30° down lens and allows for more intuitive nerve dissection toward the penis, while minimizing the risk of neuropraxic injury to the NVB (which is more likely in a retrograde approach). After ligation of the small vessels of the prostatic pedicle entering the prostate posterolaterally (as opposed to en masse ligation of the pedicle), the plane allows relatively avascular dissection (except anteriorly where the prostatic fascia merges with the venous plexus and prostate capsule). When performed correctly, an intact "veil" of periprostatic tissue extends between the pubourethral ligaments and the bladder neck. In their cohort of 154 men, 96% reported erections sufficient for intercourse (with or without PDE-5 inhibitors) at 12 months follow-up, with a PSM rate of 5% (majority of which were at the apex) [21, 22] (Fig. 1.13). Similarly, Stolzenburg et al. reported a potency rate of ~90% in patients aged <55 years old 12 months after intrafascial nerve sparing RP [28], with PSM of 4.5 and 29.4% in pT2 and pT3 disease, respectively. Nonetheless, intrafascial dissection does entail significant highest risk of PSM (at least in the beginner's hands): while significantly lower nerve bundle counts were noted in histopathological specimens after Veil nerve sparing technique (compared to standard nerve sparing), the mean margin clearance in the former specimens was just 0.3 mm (compared to 1.4 mm in the latter) [27].

Interfascial Dissection

Interfascial dissection occurs in the place outside or lateral to the prostatic fascia at the anterolateral and posterolateral aspects of the prostate, with dissection continued medial to the NVB at the 5 o' clock and 7 o' clock positions, such that the lateral and posterior surfaces of the prostate remain covered with prostatic fascia and Denonvilliers' fascia, respectively (Fig. 1.10). The classically described standard nerve sparing technique by Walsh was, in fact, an interfascial dissection. While this technique may sacrifice the periprostatic nerves distributed on the anterolateral surface of the prostate, a high anterior release modification may salvage some of these fibers (though fibers ramifying within and below the prostatic fascia will still be resected). Interfascial dissection represents a more oncologically conservative approach than the intrafascial dissection; however, at the cost of significantly inferior potency outcomes at 6 and 12 months after surgery [29, 30], and possibly even continence [29].

Extrafascial Dissection

Dissection in a plane lateral to the levator ani fascia and posterior to the Denonvilliers' fascia. The posterolateral NVB and the ventrally distributed nerve fibers, along with all the layers of prostatic, levator ani, and Denonvilliers' fascia, are resected, offering wider surgical margins but causing almost complete loss of erectile function [18] (Fig. 1.10).

Although the terms intrafascial and interfascial may help in conceptualizing the fascial anatomy around the prostate, in our opinion, there is no single fascial layer; rather, there are multiple layers (that may or may not be clearly delineated in all patients). In our experience, it is impossible to stay precisely in the same layer throughout the entire dissection. Indeed, it is not uncommon to find regions of both intra- and interfascial dissections in the same histopathological specimen.

Recognizing the importance of nerve sparing approaches in maintaining the balance between optimal functional outcomes and maximal oncologic efficacy, Tewari et al. [31] proposed a risk-stratified approach to nerve sparing ("incremental nerve sparing") according to the patient's likelihood of harboring extra-prostatic extension of PCa, as illustrated in Fig. 1.14. Similar graded nerve sparing techniques were described by Schatloff et al. (Grade 1–5, with 1 being no nerve sparing and 5 being >95 % nerve sparing) [32].

Anatomical Principles for Recovery of Urinary Continence

Despite the greater dexterity of movement and more precise dissection offered by the robotic technique, rates of urinary continence in the contemporary era remain variable, and although 12 months outcomes may be encouraging (between 84 and 97 %) [33], incontinence continues to be the most important determinant of postoperative quality of life (in some reports, even greater than erectile dysfunction). While differences in continence outcomes, much like erectile function, may stem from the multiplicity of assessment measures (number of pads/pad weights, validated questionnaires such as EPIC, ICIQ and IPSS, or patient–physician interviews), a host of

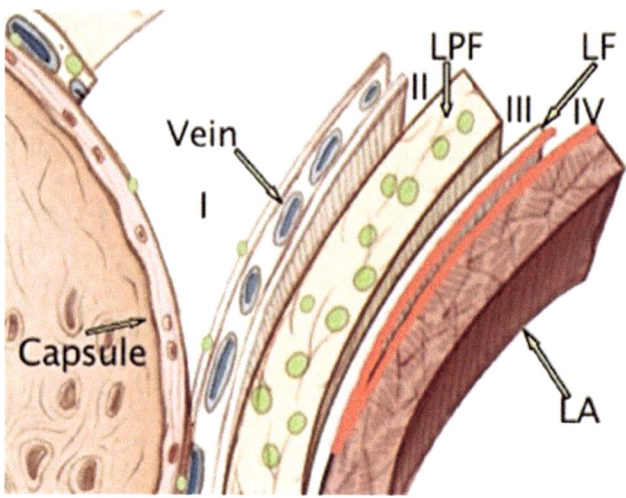

Fig. 1.14 Layers of fascia enveloping the prostatic capsule, showing the planes of dissection for differing NS grades (1–4). *LPF*, lateral pelvic fascia medial layer, i.e. the prostatic fascia; *LF*, lateral pelvic fascia lateral layer, i.e. the levator fascia; *LA*, levator ani. (From Tewari AK, Srivastava A, Huang MW, Robinson BD, Shevchuk MM, Durand M, et al. Anatomical grades of nerve sparing: a risk-stratified approach to neural-hammock sparing during robot-assisted radical prostatectomy (RARP). BJU Int. 2011 Sep;108(6 Pt 2):984–92) (Reproduced, with permission, from Wiley)

preoperative (age, BMI, preexisting lower urinary tract symptoms, and prostate size), intraoperative and postoperative factors (pelvic floor exercises, fluid intake, duration of catheterization, etc.) can also meaningfully affect the trajectory of urinary continence recovery after RARP. Intraoperative factors determining continence outcomes are based on the anatomical understanding of two main systems responsible for maintaining continence: a sphincteric system and a support system [34].

Sphincteric System

Two distinct sphincteric mechanisms control urinary continence in males. Proximally, the *internal (or vesical/preprostatic) sphincter* is derived from the ring-shaped fibers of the middle circular detrusor layer encircling the bladder neck (reinforced by the anterior collar like thickening of the outer longitudinal layer), along with the distal extension of the inner longitudinal and middle circular fiber layers from the bladder neck into the prostatic urethra up to the level of verumontanum (Fig. 1.15). The magnification provided by the robotic platform, along with the scalable movements, may help overcome the absence of tactile feedback in identifying and dissecting the bladder neck during RP. A number of maneuvers can aid in the accurate identification of the plane for bladder neck dissection: (a) Distal margin of the prevesical fat pad of Whitmore; (b) intermittent 'tugging' (caudal retraction) of the urethral catheter balloon can better delineate the point of junction between the bladder neck and prostate;

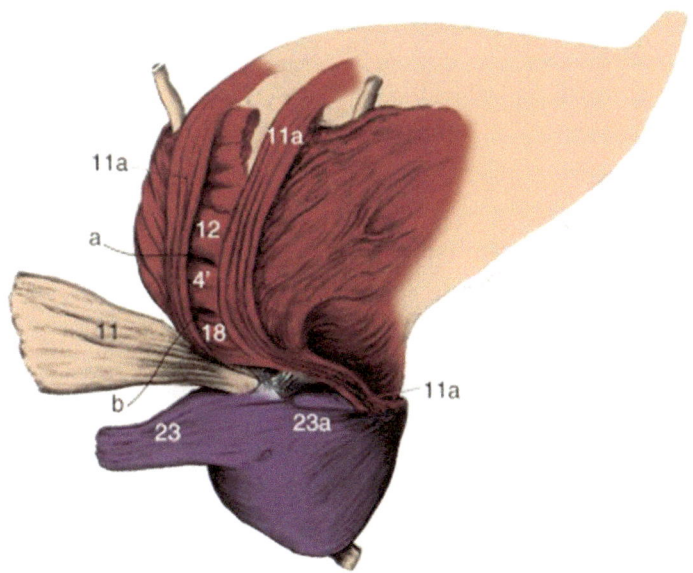

Fig. 1.15 Dissection of the male bladder. *11*, Posterior outer longitudinal detrusor, which forms the backing of the ureters (folded back); *11a*, posterolateral portion of the outer longitudinal muscle forming a loop around the anterior bladder neck; *4′*, *12*, and *18*, middle circular layer backing the trigone; *23* and *23a*, lateral pedicle of the prostate. [From Chung B, Sommer G and Brooks JD (2016). Surgical, Radiographic and Endoscopic Anatomy of the Male Pelvis. In: Wein A, Kavoussi L, Partin W and Peters C (Eds.), Campbell-Walsh Urology (pp 1611–1630). Philadelphia, PA: Elsevier] (Reproduced, with permission, from Elsevier [Campbell-Walsh urology])

(c) grasping the dome of the bladder and applying anterocephalad retraction causes 'tenting' of the bladder neck, the distal edge of which may serve as the incision point for bladder neck dissection [35]; and (d) Bimanual "palpation" or "pinch" of the bladder neck using the tips of the robotic/laparoscopic instruments [36].

Distal to the prostatic apex is the *external urethral sphincter*, formed by a complex of smooth and striated muscle fibers and surrounding the membranous urethra. The external sphincter is actually signet-ring shaped, conical structure when seen in sagittal and coronal sections, respectively, broad at its base distally and narrowing as it passes through the urogenital hiatus of the levator ani to meet the prostatic apex [37] (Fig. 1.16). The inner smooth muscular layer (subdivided into inner longitudinal and outer circular layers) of the membranous urethra is termed the *lissosphincter* by some authors. Conversely, the outer muscle layer is termed the *rhabdosphincter* and is horseshoe or omega shaped in cross section (Fig. 1.6). Anteriorly and anterolaterally, these fibers insert on the apex and the anterior surface of the prostate, with attachments to the subpubic fascia and medial fascia of the levator ani, and merge posteriorly with the tendinous midline dorsal raphe (MDR), a musculofascial plate that extends along the entire length of the rhabdosphincer along its dorsal aspect. The external sphincter is innervated by autonomic branches of pelvic plexus, which

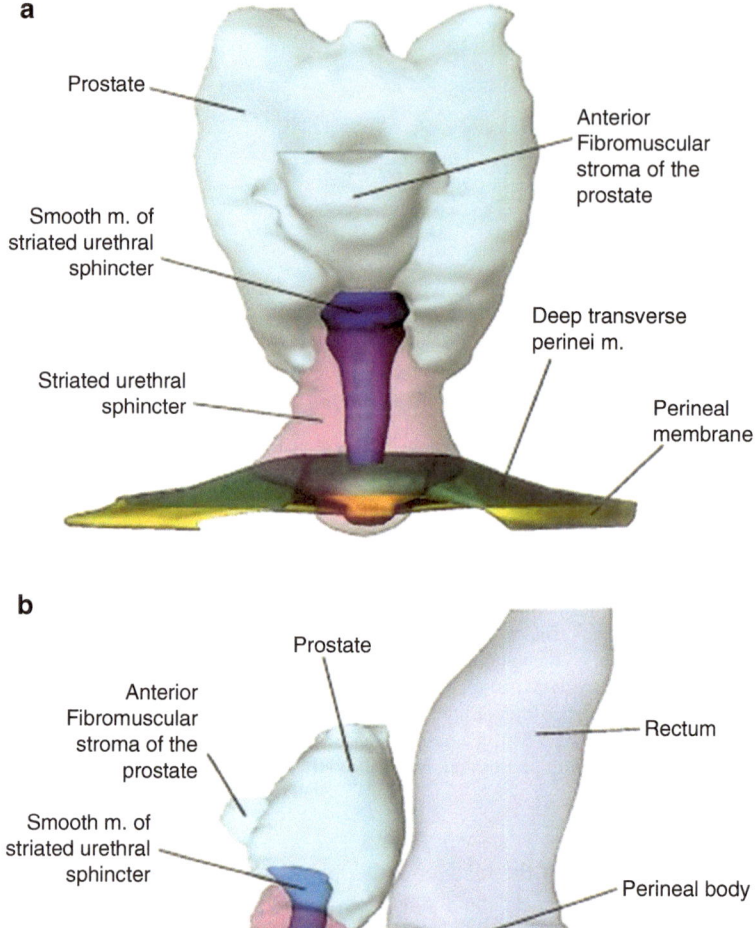

Fig. 1.16 Structure of the male striated urethral sphincter. (**a**) Anterior projection shows the cone shape of the sphincter and the smooth muscle of the sphincter. (**b**) Viewed laterally, the anterior wall of the sphincter is nearly twice the length of the posterior wall, although both are of comparable thickness. [From Chung B, Sommer G and Brooks JD (2016). Surgical, Radiographic and Endoscopic Anatomy of the Male Pelvis. In: Wein A, Kavoussi L, Partin W and Peters C (Eds.), Campbell-Walsh Urology (pp 1611–1630). Philadelphia, PA: Elsevier] (Reproduced, with permission, from Elsevier [Campbell-Walsh urology])

run partly with the NVB and partly with the perineal branch of pudendal nerve. Nerves enter the sphincter posterolaterally, mainly concentrated on the 5 and 7 o' clock positions. Muscle fibers in the striated layer are mostly slow twitch (type 1) fibers, which are responsible for maintaining a constant tone for passive urinary control, as well as allowing voluntary increases in tone to provide additional continence protection [37].

An important structure in close relation to the external sphincter is the dorsal vascular complex (DVC) or the eponymously termed Santorini's plexus. It drains venous blood from the deep dorsal vein of the penis, trifurcating at the prostatourethral junction by the presence of PPLs into a central superficial branch (which pierces the endopelvic fascia between the PPLs and drains the retropubic fat, anterior bladder, and anterior prostate) and a deeper trunk (which remains deep to the endopelvic and prostatic fascia and sweeps upward and laterally to drain blood from the periprostatic plexus, rectum, and the vesical plexus to continue as inferior vesical veins) [38]. Therefore, Walsh suggested ligation and division of the DVC be done distally before its ramification, in order to avoid blood loss and compromised vision during radical retropubic prostatectomy [38]. Additionally, at this level, the DVC is separated from the rhabdosphincter by the rhabdosphincter fascia; this provides an avascular plane for dissection and DVC control (Fig. 1.6). Part of the DVC, however, may run within the substance of the external sphincter, necessitating careful dissection when attempting to secure hemostasis. As such, preservation or selective ligation of the DVC may hasten return to urinary continence [38] (see later).

Embryologically, the rhabdosphincter exists as a continuous, vertically oriented tube from the bladder neck to the perineal membrane: as the prostate grows into it, it causes atrophy of the muscular mass. This has important implications with reference to variations in apical anatomy (Fig. 1.17): Myers et al. [39] and Lee et al. [40] have shown that the apex may overlap the striated sphincter circumferentially, asymmetrically bilaterally or unilaterally, anteriorly, posteriorly, or no overlap with the sphincter (in descending order of frequency). This needs to be kept in mind during apical dissection, in order to prevent inadvertent excessive resection of the sphincteric tissue and compromising postoperative membranous urethral length.

Supportive System

The key supportive structures in the normal (preprostatectomy) male are shown in Fig. 1.18 [34]. From anterior to posterior, these structures include the pubovesical/puboprostatic ligaments (PV/PPLs), the endopelvic fascia, FTAP, levator ani musculature, and the Denonvilliers' fascia.

The PV/PPLs are paired fibrocollagenous extensions of the visceral endopelvic fascia that extend from the anteroinferior surface of the prostate and the anterior surface of the urethral sphincter, to the periosteum over the posteroinferior surface of the pubis bone. These ligamentous structures support the bladder, prostate, and

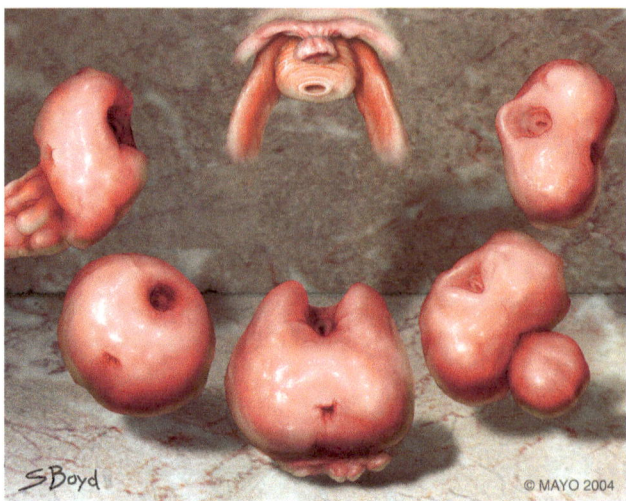

Fig. 1.17 Variations in apical shapes of prostates. Started from left, the apex can overlap the urethral sphincter anteriorly, circumferentially, symmetrically bilaterally, asymmetrically unilaterally, or posteriorly with anterior apical notch and posterior lip. (From Walz J, Burnett AL, Costello AJ, Eastham JA, Graefen M, Guillonneau B, et al. A critical analysis of the current knowledge of surgical anatomy related to optimization of cancer control and preservation of continence and erection in candidates for radical prostatectomy. Eur Urol. 2010 Feb;57(2):179–92) (Reproduced, with permission, from Elsevier)

the external sphincter and help "suspend" the internal and external sphincter within the pelvic cavity. The two leaves of the endopelvic fascia (parietal and visceral), along with their line of fusion (FTAP), form a part of continuous scaffolding that extends anteriorly from the PV/PPLs to the ischial spine.

The floor of the pelvic cavity is bounded anteriorly by the levator ani muscle, formed by the fibers of pubococcygeus anteriorly and iliococcygeus posteriorly. Close to the urogenital hiatus, the fibers of levator ani are thickened to flank the prostatoturethral junction, spanning from the pubis anteriorly to the perineal body posteriorly, and is known as puboperinealis [41, 42]. Composed predominantly of fast twitch (type 2) fibers, contraction of the puboperinealis muscle closes off the urethral lumen and actively terminates micturition. Further, while the contraction of puboperinealis pulls the urethra upward and forward toward the pubis bone, contraction of the rhabdosphincter pulls it downward and backward toward the perineal body (with the posterior musculofascial plate acting as the fulcrum for the movement of the rhabdosphincter). This causes a double-sling mechanism for closing the urethra and hence maintaining continence [41, 43]. The role of the supportive mechanism is, therefore, to support the bladder, prostate, and the external sphincter within the pelvic cavity: when intra-abdominal pressure increases, these structures prevent descent of proximal and distal sphincteric mechanisms (urethral hypermobility) and maintain the angulation of the vesico-prostatic junction, while contraction of the levator ani supports them from below and closes off the urethral lumen.

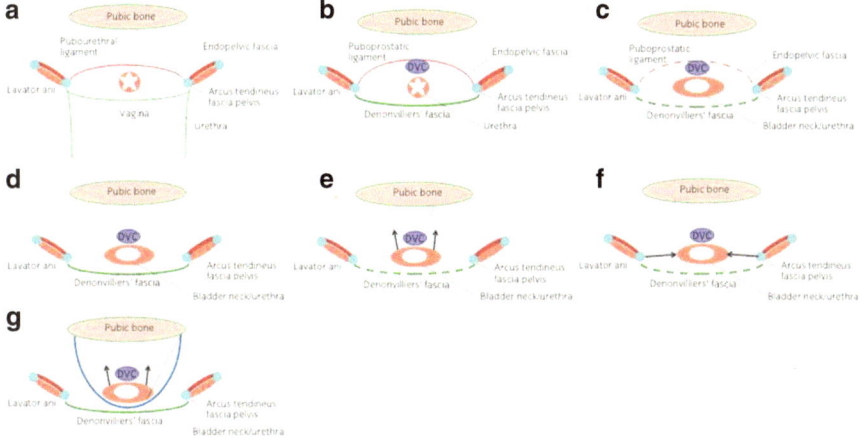

Fig. 1.18 Supporting system in the pelvis, and reconstruction and reinforcement during RARP. (**a**) Structural support in the female pelvis. (**b**) Structural support in the male pelvis. (**c**) Structural changes after radical prostatectomy. (**d**) Posterior reconstruction of the rhabdosphincter. (**e**) Anterior retropubic suspension. (**f**) Reattachment of the arcus tendineus to the bladder neck. (**g**) Bone-anchored bladder neck sling suspension. *DVC* dorsal vein complex. (From Kojima Y, Takahashi N, Haga N, Nomiya M, Yanagida T, Ishibashi K, et al. Urinary incontinence after robot-assisted radical prostatectomy: pathophysiology and intraoperative techniques to improve surgical outcome. Int J Urol. 2013 Nov;20(11):1052–63) (Reproduced, with permission, from Wiley)

Intraoperative Strategies to Promote Recovery of Urinary Continence

Components of both the sphincteric system and supportive system play varying roles in maintaining urinary continence. As such, during radical prostatectomy, it would be ideal to preserve as much of the natural pelvic anatomy as possible. In many cases, however (such as an enlarged prostate or presence of pelvic adhesions), safe preservation of structures may be precluded, and reconstruction of the natural mechanism may then be attempted to restore normal anatomy and promote continence. Accordingly, the "preserve when you can, reconstruct when you can't" strategy may be understood in Table 1.2. Detailed description of the technical details of each of these approaches is beyond the scope of this chapter; however, we attempt to provide a somewhat overarching framework for understanding the maneuvers for faster recovery of urinary continence.

Conclusions

1. The precise location and functional anatomy of the neurovascular bundle remains conjectural. The prevailing evidence suggests that there is a network of nerves that innervates the cavernous bodies, rather than discrete neurovascular bundles.

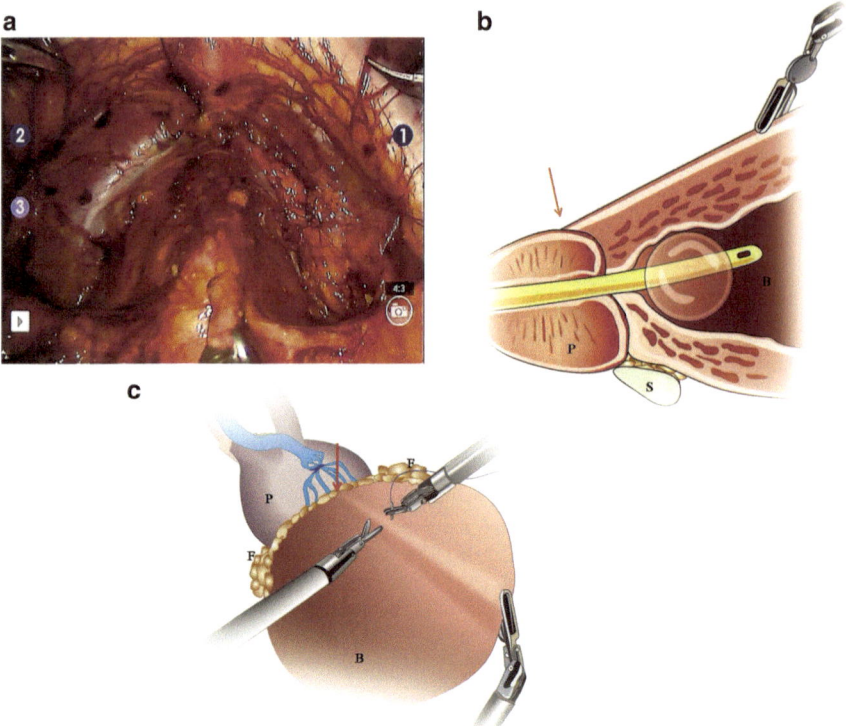

Fig. 1.19 (**a**) Anterior aspect of the vesicoprostatic junction with application of anterocephalad fourth arm Prograsp tension; (**b**) diagram of the vesicoprostatic junction; (**c**) three-dimensional view of the vesicoprostatic junction. *Red arrow* represents the point at which the tented bladder fold ends and incision is made to begin bladder neck preservation technique anteriorly. *P* prostate, *B* bladder, *S* seminal vesicle, *F* fat pad of Whitmore. (From Freire MP, Weinberg AC, Lei Y, Soukup JR, Lipsitz SR, Prasad SM, et al. Anatomic bladder neck preservation during robotic-assisted laparoscopic radical prostatectomy: description of technique and outcomes. Eur Urol. 2009 Dec;56(6):972–80) (Reproduced, with permission, from Elsevier)

In the only study that directly traced the course of periprostatic nerve fibers to the end organ (the cavernosal bodies) [25], the findings were unexpected. The posterolateral nerves appeared to innervate the corpus spongiosum, whereas cavernosal innervation was derived from nerve fibers located anterolaterally at the prostatic apex. As such, more definitive studies are needed before this controversy is settled. At the very least, given the distribution of nerve fibers along the entire surface of the prostate, it may be safe to presume that the term "neurovascular bundle" itself may be a misnomer, since neither the nerves form a distinct bundle nor do they always follow the vessels. It is easy to preserve the vessels, and by inference the nerves that lie in the proximity, yet we have amply seen (and as the subsequent chapters will show) that this does not guarantee the maintenance of erectile function.

Table 1.2 Intraoperative strategies for faster recovery of urinary continence post robot-assisted radical prostatectomy

Sphincteric mechanism	
Preservation	
Maneuver/technical modification	Results
Bladder neck (proximal sphincter) preservation (BNP)	
Friere et al. [35]: Anterocephalad tension on the bladder using the fourth robotic arm retracts the anterior dome of the bladder and forms a ridge that ends distally at the detrusor apron: landmark for incision point for bladder neck dissection (Fig. 1.19)	348 men with BNP RARP and 271 with standard RARP, higher EPIC urinary function score at 4 months (64.6 vs. 57.2; $p=0.04$), 12 months (80.6 vs. 79) and 24 months (94.1 vs. 86.8; $p<0.001$), respectively. PSM at prostate base comparable (1.4 % vs. 2.2 %)
Nyarangi-Dix et al. [44]: Blunt dissection to separate the ring-shaped vesical sphincter from prostate base and identification of longitudinal smooth muscle fibers of urethra	Randomized controlled trial: At 0, 3, 6, and 12 months mean urine loss in the control vs. BNP group was significantly lower in the latter (each $p<0.001$). Social continence rate was 55.3 % vs. 84.2 % ($p<0.001$), 74.8 % vs. 89.5 % ($p=0.05$), and 81.4 % vs. 94.7 % ($p<0.027$) at 3, 6, and 12 months
Rhabdosphincter (external sphincter) preservation	
Selective suture ligation of DVC (Walsh)	
Laparoscopic RP (Porpiglia et al. [45]): Prior to urethral transection, insufflation pressure increased to 16–18 mmHg and DVC sectioned. Following urethral transection and prostate excision, SSL performed with one/two stitches in figure-of-8 fashion avoiding entry into rhabdosphincter	Higher urinary continence in SSL vs. standard laparoscopic RP at 3 months (80 % vs. 53 %; $p=0.02$), although no difference at 6 or 12 months. No significant difference in apical PSM
RARP (Lei et al. [46]): Selective mattress suturing is performed after cold scissor transection of the DVC, followed by urethrovesical anastomosis. Pneumoperitoneum ensures hemostasis, and SSL minimizes injury to the rhabdosphincter as well as levator ani	SSL vs. standard RARP had significantly higher 5-month postoperative urinary function score and continence, and independently predicted better urinary function score recovery of continence 5 months post-RARP
Maximizing functional urethral length	
Tewari et al. [47]: Identification of the prostatourethral junction, followed by incision on the posterior hemicircumference of urethra. Anterior wall clearly visible, and circumferential urethral division using blunt and sharp dissection	Significantly lower apical PSM compared to the control group (1.4 % vs. 4.4 %, $p=0.04$), despite higher proportion of pT3a or higher disease in the former group (16 % vs. 10 %, $p=0.027$)
Schlomm et al. [48]: Full-functional urethral length preservation according to the patient's anatomy: careful preservation of the puboperinealis muscle fibers and restoration of the Mueller's ligaments (ischioprostatic ligaments)	406 patients with full urethral length preserving RP had higher continence at 1 week than 285 patients with conventional RP (50.1 % vs. 30.9 %, respectively, $p<0.001$). Only independent predictor of 1-week continence status

(continued)

Table 1.2 (continued)

Nerve preservation	
Choi et al. [49]: Comparison of outcomes for bilateral vs. nonnerve sparing (NS)	Both EPIC urinary function score and continence rates higher in bilateral NS vs. non-NS at 4 months, but only urinary function scores higher at 12 and 24 months
Stolzenburg et al. [29]: Randomized controlled trial between intrafascial and interfascial nerve-sparing endoscopic extra peritoneal RP (EERPE)	Intrafascial vs. interfascial EERPE had significantly higher continence at 3 months (74 % vs. 63 %) and 6 months (87.9 % vs. 76.2 %), respectively (both $p < 0.05$)
Steineck et al. [50]: LAPPRO steering committee performed multicentric study, comparing urinary continence after varying degrees of nerve preservation	Compared to bilateral intrafascial dissection (reference category, relative risk [RR] = 1), decreasing levels of nerve preservation associated with decreasing likelihood of urinary continence at 1 year, with no NVB preservation having a RR = 2.27. Similar trends noted in men with preoperative impotence, urinary incontinence, open and robotic RP
Reeves et al. [51]: Meta-analyses of studies on NVB preservation and urinary continence recovery	Patients with any NS surgery (uni or bilateral) had significantly better early continence vs. those with non-NS surgery at 6 weeks, 3–4 months and 6 months (RR 1.48, 1.24, and 1.20 respectively), but no significant differences at 12 or 24 months. Similar results when comparing bilateral to unilateral NS surgery
Michl et al. [52]: Comparison of urinary continence outcomes for bilateral NS RP, primary non-NS RP, and bilateral secondary resection of the NVBs for positive frozen section results after an initial bilateral NS sparing (secNNS) RP	Continence rates at 12 months after surgery did not differ significantly between patients who had bilateral NS and secNNS (85.4 % vs. 87.0 %). Conversely, for initial NNS versus secNNS, the latter group had significantly higher continence rates after 12 months (70.5 % vs. 87.0 %). Authors conclude that meticulous apical dissection performed during NS RP technique is responsible for higher continence rates rather than the actual preservation of the NVB itself
Reconstruction	
Maneuver/technical modification	Results
Bladder neck (BN) reconstruction	
Lin et al. [53]: Transverse plication of anterior BN in RARP patients	97.3 % men were fully continent (0 pad/day) at 12 months after surgery
Lee et al. [54]: Compared RARP patients with transverse plication of BN to historical controls without BN plication	Mean time to social continence (0–1 pad/day) in plication vs. standard group 3.6 vs. 5.3 weeks (p-0.004) and total continence (0 pad/day) 5.1 vs. 8.5 weeks ($p = 0.002$)

(continued)

Table 1.2 (continued)

Supportive mechanism	
Preservation	
Puboprostatic ligaments	
Stolzenburg et al. [55]	PPL sparing vs. conventional RARP continence at 2 weeks (24 % vs. 12 %) and 4 weeks (76 % and 48 %), respectively (*p* < 0.05)
Puboprostatic collar	
Tewari et al. [56]: Preservation of puboprostatic ligaments, puboperinealis muscle, and arcus tendineus (together called the puboprostatic collar)	Urinary continence rates at 1, 6, 12, and 16 weeks were 29, 62, 88, and 95 %; no differences in perioperative, functional, or oncologic outcomes
Pubovesical complex sparing (complete anterior preservation)	
Asimakopoulos et al. [57]: Owing to the anatomic continuity between puboprostatic ligaments with detrusor apron, preservation of the entire pubovesical complex (DVC, puboprostatic ligaments, and detrusor apron) attempted in 30 preoperatively healthy and continent men	Urinary continence was 80 % at catheter removal and 100 % at 3 months after surgery
Bocciardi et al. [58, 59]: Retzius sparing prostatectomy performed through incision on the pouch of Douglas. Allows for preservation of the pubovesical complex, levator ani, arcus tendineus, and anterior fixation of the bladder to the abdominal wall	Immediate social continence rates (i.e., on removal of catheter) was 91 %, and 1 year continence was 96 %
Menon et al. (unpublished data): Retzius sparing prostatectomy (RSP)	4-week total continence rates for RSP vs. VIP 79 % vs. 36 %, respectively; 4 week social continence 95.1 % vs. 61.0 %, respectively (both *p* < 0.001)
Reconstruction	
Periurethral suspension stitch (anterior reconstruction)	
Noguchi et al. [60]: Reversal of the DVC suture through the symphysis pubis perichondrium during open retropubic RP	Shorter median time to recovery of urinary continence in suspension stitch vs. standard group (31 vs. 90 days; *p* = 0.002)
Patel et al. [61]: Periurethral retropubic suspension stitch, from DVC to the periosteum of the pubic bone, in a figure-of-8 fashion, done following DVC ligation	Shorter median time to recovery of urinary continence in suspension stitch vs. standard group (6 weeks vs. 7 weeks; *p* = 0.02). Significantly higher continence rates at 3 months (92.8 vs. 83 %)
Posterior reconstruction (PR) of the rhabdosphincter and Denonvilliers' musculofascial plate	

(continued)

Table 1.2 (continued)

Rocco et al. [62]: Reconstruction of the posterior musculofascial plate by suturing the dorsal median raphe of the rhabdosphincter to the remnant of the Denonvilliers' fascia posterior to the bladder; the newly created Denonvilliers' plate is then attached to the posterior bladder wall. Restores the functional and anatomical sphincter length, supports the posterior aspect of the external urethral sphincter and urethrovesical anastomoses, and avoids caudal retraction of the urethro-sphincteric complex	PR group had significantly higher continence than historical controls: 72% vs. 14%, 78.8% vs. 30%, and 86% vs. 46% at 3, 30, and 90 days, respectively
Joshi et al. [63]: Randomized controlled trial comparing RARP with vs. without PR ($n=54$ each)	Urinary continence for PR vs. standard RARP at 3 months (25 and 31%) and 6 months (49% vs. 57%), respectively; no significant difference
Combined anterior and posterior reconstruction	
Menon et al. [64]: RCT comparing AR plus PR vs. standard RARP ($n=57$ each)	No significant difference in social (0–1 pad/day) or total continence (0 pad/day) at 1, 2, 7, and 30 days (all $p>0.1$). 1 m social and total continence rates for intervention vs. standard RARP were (80% vs. 74%) and (47% vs. 42%), respectively
Sammon et al. [65]: Long-term follow-up of previous RCT patients	No differences between groups regarding urine leakage weights, pad usage rates, long-term IPSS score, or IPSS bother score. 12–24 months total continence rates for AR+PR vs. Standard RARP group 83 and 80%, respectively
Hurtes et al. [66]: RCT comparing AR plus PR vs. standard RARP	Total continence rates for intervention vs. control groups were 26.5 and 7.1% at 1 months ($p=0.047$), 45.2 and 15.4% at 3 months ($p=0.016$). No significant difference at 6 months
Total anatomical reconstruction of vesicourethral junction	
Tewari et al. [67]: Minimal distal incision of the endopelvic fascia, preservation of the puboperinealis, preservation of PPL, watertight urethrovesical anastomosis, reattachment of the arcus tendineus to the lateral aspect of the bladder neck	Continence rates were 38, 83, 91, and 97% at 1, 6, 12, 24 weeks, respectively

2. Preservation of urinary continence is much more predictable. Factors associated with earlier return of urinary control are "no-touch" apical dissection, preservation of the bladder neck, and maximal nerve preservation. A surgical approach preserving the Retzius space may improve these results in the majority of patients.

Acknowledgment *Financial disclosures and conflicts of interest*: None.

References

1. Rogers CG, Trock BP, Walsh PC. Preservation of accessory pudendal arteries during radical retropubic prostatectomy: surgical technique and results. Urology. 2004;64(1):148–51.
2. Rosen MP, Greenfield AJ, Walker TG, Grant P, Guben JK, Dubrow J, et al. Arteriogenic impotence: findings in 195 impotent men examined with selective internal pudendal angiography. Young Investigator's Award. Radiology. 1990;174(3 Pt 2):1043–8.
3. Muller J. Über die organischen Nerven der erectilen männlichen Geschlectsorgane des Menschen und der Säugethiere [concerning the autonomic nerves of the male erectile genital organs of man and mammals]. Berlin: F. Dummler; 1836.
4. Finkle AL, Saunders JB. Sexual potency in aging males. III. Technic of avoiding nerve injury in perineal prostatic operations. Am J Surg. 1960;99:23–6.
5. Schlegel PN, Walsh PC. Neuroanatomical approach to radical cystoprostatectomy with preservation of sexual function. J Urol. 1987;138(6):1402–6.
6. Walsh PC, Donker PJ. Impotence following radical prostatectomy: insight into etiology and prevention. J Urol. 1982;128(3):492–7.
7. Walsh PC, Lepor H, Eggleston JC. Radical prostatectomy with preservation of sexual function: anatomical and pathological considerations. Prostate. 1983;4(5):473–85.
8. Menon M, Shrivastava A, Tewari A, Sarle R, Hemal A, Peabody JO, et al. Laparoscopic and robot assisted radical prostatectomy: establishment of a structured program and preliminary analysis of outcomes. J Urol. 2002;168(3):945–9.
9. Tewari A, Peabody JO, Fischer M, Sarle R, Vallancien G, Delmas V, et al. An operative and anatomic study to help in nerve sparing during laparoscopic and robotic radical prostatectomy. Eur Urol. 2003;43(5):444–54.
10. Costello AJ, Brooks M, Cole OJ. Anatomical studies of the neurovascular bundle and cavernosal nerves. BJU Int. 2004;94(7):1071–6.
11. Kourambas J, Angus DG, Hosking P, Chou ST. A histological study of Denonvilliers' fascia and its relationship to the neurovascular bundle. Br J Urol. 1998;82(3):408–10.
12. Kiyoshima K, Yokomizo A, Yoshida T, Tomita K, Yonemasu H, Nakamura M, et al. Anatomical features of periprostatic tissue and its surroundings: a histological analysis of 79 radical retropubic prostatectomy specimens. Jpn J Clin Oncol. 2004;34(8):463–8.
13. Takenaka A, Murakami G, Soga H, Han SH, Arai Y, Fujisawa M. Anatomical analysis of the neurovascular bundle supplying penile cavernous tissue to ensure a reliable nerve graft after radical prostatectomy. J Urol. 2004;172(3):1032–5.
14. Lunacek A, Schwentner C, Fritsch H, Bartsch G, Strasser H. Anatomical radical retropubic prostatectomy: 'curtain dissection' of the neurovascular bundle. BJU Int. 2005;95(9):1226–31.
15. Eichelberg C, Erbersdobler A, Michl U, Schlomm T, Salomon G, Graefen M, et al. Nerve distribution along the prostatic capsule. Eur Urol. 2007;51(1):105–10. discussion 10-1.
16. Tewari A, Takenaka A, Mtui E, Horninger W, Peschel R, Bartsch G, et al. The proximal neurovascular plate and the tri-zonal neural architecture around the prostate gland: importance in the athermal robotic technique of nerve-sparing prostatectomy. BJU Int. 2006;98(2):314–23.
17. Ganzer R, Blana A, Gaumann A, Stolzenburg JU, Rabenalt R, Bach T, et al. Topographical anatomy of periprostatic and capsular nerves: quantification and computerised planimetry. Eur Urol. 2008;54(2):353–60.
18. Walz J, Burnett AL, Costello AJ, Eastham JA, Graefen M, Guillonneau B, et al. A critical analysis of the current knowledge of surgical anatomy related to optimization of cancer control and preservation of continence and erection in candidates for radical prostatectomy. Eur Urol. 2010;57(2):179–92.
19. Montorsi F, Salonia A, Suardi N, Gallina A, Zanni G, Briganti A, et al. Improving the preservation of the urethral sphincter and neurovascular bundles during open radical retropubic prostatectomy. Eur Urol. 2005;48(6):938–45.
20. Costello AJ, Dowdle BW, Namdarian B, Pedersen J, Murphy DG. Immunohistochemical study of the cavernous nerves in the periprostatic region. BJU Int. 2011;107(8):1210–5.

21. Kaul S, Bhandari A, Hemal A, Savera A, Shrivastava A, Menon M. Robotic radical prostatectomy with preservation of the prostatic fascia: a feasibility study. Urology. 2005;66(6):1261–5.

22. Menon M, Kaul S, Bhandari A, Shrivastava A, Tewari A, Hemal A. Potency following robotic radical prostatectomy: a questionnaire based analysis of outcomes after conventional nerve sparing and prostatic fascia sparing techniques. J Urol. 2005;174(6):2291–6. discussion 6.

23. Nielsen ME, Schaeffer EM, Marschke P, Walsh PC. High anterior release of the levator fascia improves sexual function following open radical retropubic prostatectomy. J Urol. 2008;180(6):2557–64. discussion 64.

24. Hubanks JM, Umbreit EC, Karnes RJ, Myers RP. Open radical retropubic prostatectomy using high anterior release of the levator fascia and constant haptic feedback in bilateral neurovascular bundle preservation plus early postoperative phosphodiesterase type 5 inhibition: a contemporary series. Eur Urol. 2012;61(5):878–84.

25. Alsaid B, Bessede T, Diallo D, Moszkowicz D, Karam I, Benoit G, et al. Division of autonomic nerves within the neurovascular bundles distally into corpora cavernosa and corpus spongiosum components: immunohistochemical confirmation with three-dimensional reconstruction. Eur Urol. 2011;59(6):902–9.

26. Villers A, McNeal JE, Freiha FS, Boccon-Gibod L, Stamey TA. Invasion of Denonvilliers' fascia in radical prostatectomy specimens. J Urol. 1993;149(4):793–8.

27. Savera AT, Kaul S, Badani K, Stark AT, Shah NL, Menon M. Robotic radical prostatectomy with the "Veil of Aphrodite" technique: histologic evidence of enhanced nerve sparing. Eur Urol. 2006;49(6):1065–73. discussion 73-4.

28. Stolzenburg JU, Rabenalt R, Do M, Schwalenberg T, Winkler M, Dietel A, et al. Intrafascial nerve-sparing endoscopic extraperitoneal radical prostatectomy. Eur Urol. 2008; 53(5):931–40.

29. Stolzenburg JU, Kallidonis P, Do M, Dietel A, Hafner T, Rabenalt R, et al. A comparison of outcomes for interfascial and intrafascial nerve-sparing radical prostatectomy. Urology. 2010;76(3):743–8.

30. Zheng T, Zhang X, Ma X, Li HZ, Gao JP, Cai W, et al. A matched-pair comparison between bilateral intrafascial and interfascial nerve-sparing techniques in extraperitoneal laparoscopic radical prostatectomy. Asian J Androl. 2013;15(4):513–7.

31. Tewari AK, Srivastava A, Huang MW, Robinson BD, Shevchuk MM, Durand M, et al. Anatomical grades of nerve sparing: a risk-stratified approach to neural-hammock sparing during robot-assisted radical prostatectomy (RARP). BJU Int. 2011;108(6 Pt 2):984–92.

32. Schatloff O, Chauhan S, Sivaraman A, Kameh D, Palmer KJ, Patel VR. Anatomic grading of nerve sparing during robot-assisted radical prostatectomy. Eur Urol. 2012;61(4):796–802.

33. Ficarra V, Novara G, Rosen RC, Artibani W, Carroll PR, Costello A, et al. Systematic review and meta-analysis of studies reporting urinary continence recovery after robot-assisted radical prostatectomy. Eur Urol. 2012;62(3):405–17.

34. Kojima Y, Takahashi N, Haga N, Nomiya M, Yanagida T, Ishibashi K, et al. Urinary incontinence after robot-assisted radical prostatectomy: pathophysiology and intraoperative techniques to improve surgical outcome. Int J Urol. 2013;20(11):1052–63.

35. Freire MP, Weinberg AC, Lei Y, Soukup JR, Lipsitz SR, Prasad SM, et al. Anatomic bladder neck preservation during robotic-assisted laparoscopic radical prostatectomy: description of technique and outcomes. Eur Urol. 2009;56(6):972–80.

36. Li-Ming S, Smith J. Laparoscopic and Robotic-assisted Laparoscopic Radical Prostatectomy and Pelvic Lymphadenectomy. In: Kavoussi L, Novick A, Partin A, Peters C, editors. Campbell-Walsh urology. Philadelphia, PA: Elsevier; 2012.

37. Chung B, Sommer G, Brooks J. Anatomy of the Lower Urinary Tract and Male Genitalia. In: Kavoussi L, Novick A, Partin A, Peters C, editors. Campbell-Walsh urology. Philadelphia, PA: Elsevier; 2012.

38. Schaeffer E, Partin A, Lepor H, Walsh PC. Radical Retropubic and Perineal Prostatectomy. In: Kavoussi L, Novick A, Partin A, Peters C, editors. Campbell-Walsh urology. Philadelphia, PA: Elsevier; 2012.

39. Myers RP, Villers A. Anatomic considerations in radical prostatectomy. In: Kirby R, Partin A, Feneley M, Parsons J, editors. Prostate cancer; principle and practice. Abingdon: Taylor & Francis; 2006. p. 701–13.

40. Lee SE, Byun SS, Lee HJ, Song SH, Chang IH, Kim YJ, et al. Impact of variations in prostatic apex shape on early recovery of urinary continence after radical retropubic prostatectomy. Urology. 2006;68(1):137–41.

41. Myers RP, Cahill DR, Kay PA, Camp JJ, Devine RM, King BF, et al. Puboperineales: muscular boundaries of the male urogenital hiatus in 3D from magnetic resonance imaging. J Urol. 2000;164(4):1412–5.

42. Brooks JD, Chao WM, Kerr J. Male pelvic anatomy reconstructed from the visible human data set. J Urol. 1998;159(3):868–72.

43. Strasser H, Klima G, Poisel S, Horninger W, Bartsch G. Anatomy and innervation of the rhabdosphincter of the male urethra. Prostate. 1996;28(1):24–31.

44. Nyarangi-Dix JN, Radtke JP, Hadaschik B, Pahernik S, Hohenfellner M. Impact of complete bladder neck preservation on urinary continence, quality of life and surgical margins after radical prostatectomy: a randomized, controlled, single blind trial. J Urol. 2013;189(3):891–8.

45. Porpiglia F, Fiori C, Grande S, Morra I, Scarpa RM. Selective versus standard ligature of the deep venous complex during laparoscopic radical prostatectomy: effects on continence, blood loss, and margin status. Eur Urol. 2009;55(6):1377–83.

46. Lei Y, Alemozaffar M, Williams SB, Hevelone N, Lipsitz SR, Plaster BA, et al. Athermal division and selective suture ligation of the dorsal vein complex during robot-assisted laparoscopic radical prostatectomy: description of technique and outcomes. Eur Urol. 2011;59(2):235–43.

47. Tewari AK, Srivastava A, Mudaliar K, Tan GY, Grover S, El Douaihy Y, et al. Anatomical retro-apical technique of synchronous (posterior and anterior) urethral transection: a novel approach for ameliorating apical margin positivity during robotic radical prostatectomy. BJU Int. 2010;106(9):1364–73.

48. Schlomm T, Heinzer H, Steuber T, Salomon G, Engel O, Michl U, et al. Full functional-length urethral sphincter preservation during radical prostatectomy. Eur Urol. 2011;60(2):320–9.

49. Choi WW, Freire MP, Soukup JR, Yin L, Lipsitz SR, Carvas F, et al. Nerve-sparing technique and urinary control after robot-assisted laparoscopic prostatectomy. World J Urol. 2011;29(1):21–7.

50. Steineck G, Bjartell A, Hugosson J, Axen E, Carlsson S, Stranne J, et al. Degree of preservation of the neurovascular bundles during radical prostatectomy and urinary continence 1 year after surgery. Eur Urol. 2015;67(3):559–68.

51. Reeves F, Preece P, Kapoor J, Everaerts W, Murphy DG, Corcoran NM, et al. Preservation of the neurovascular bundles is associated with improved time to continence after radical prostatectomy but not long-term continence rates: results of a systematic review and meta-analysis. Eur Urol. 2015;68(4):692–704.

52. Michl U, Tennstedt P, Feldmeier L, Mandel P, Oh SJ, Ahyai S, et al. Nerve-sparing surgery technique, not the preservation of the neurovascular bundles, leads to improved long-term continence rates after radical prostatectomy. Eur Urol. 2016;69(4):584–9.

53. Lin VC, Coughlin G, Savamedi S, Palmer KJ, Coelho RF, Patel VR. Modified transverse plication for bladder neck reconstruction during robotic-assisted laparoscopic prostatectomy. BJU Int. 2009;104(6):878–81.

54. Lee DI, Wedmid A, Mendoza P, Sharma S, Walicki M, Hastings R, et al. Bladder neck plication stitch: a novel technique during robot-assisted radical prostatectomy to improve recovery of urinary continence. J Endourol. 2011;25(12):1873–7.

55. Stolzenburg JU, Liatsikos EN, Rabenalt R, Do M, Sakelaropoulos G, Horn LC, et al. Nerve sparing endoscopic extraperitoneal radical prostatectomy—effect of puboprostatic ligament preservation on early continence and positive margins. Eur Urol. 2006;49(1):103–11. discussion 11-2.

56. Tewari AK, Bigelow K, Rao S, Takenaka A, El-Tabi N, Te A, et al. Anatomic restoration technique of continence mechanism and preservation of puboprostatic collar: a novel modification to achieve early urinary continence in men undergoing robotic prostatectomy. Urology. 2007;69(4):726–31.

57. Asimakopoulos AD, Annino F, D'Orazio A, Pereira CF, Mugnier C, Hoepffner JL, et al. Complete periprostatic anatomy preservation during robot-assisted laparoscopic radical prostatectomy (RALP): the new pubovesical complex-sparing technique. Eur Urol. 2010; 58(3):407–17.
58. Galfano A, Ascione A, Grimaldi S, Petralia G, Strada E, Bocciardi AM. A new anatomic approach for robot-assisted laparoscopic prostatectomy: a feasibility study for completely intrafascial surgery. Eur Urol. 2010;58(3):457–61.
59. Galfano A, Di Trapani D, Sozzi F, Strada E, Petralia G, Bramerio M, et al. Beyond the learning curve of the Retzius-sparing approach for robot-assisted laparoscopic radical prostatectomy: oncologic and functional results of the first 200 patients with >/= 1 year of follow-up. Eur Urol. 2013;64(6):974–80.
60. Noguchi M, Kakuma T, Suekane S, Nakashima O, Mohamed ER, Matsuoka K. A randomized clinical trial of suspension technique for improving early recovery of urinary continence after radical retropubic prostatectomy. BJU Int. 2008;102(8):958–63.
61. Patel VR, Coelho RF, Palmer KJ, Rocco B. Periurethral suspension stitch during robot-assisted laparoscopic radical prostatectomy: description of the technique and continence outcomes. Eur Urol. 2009;56(3):472–8.
62. Rocco F, Carmignani L, Acquati P, Gadda F, Dell'Orto P, Rocco B, et al. Restoration of posterior aspect of rhabdosphincter shortens continence time after radical retropubic prostatectomy. J Urol. 2006;175(6):2201–6.
63. Joshi N, de Blok W, van Muilekom E, van der Poel H. Impact of posterior musculofascial reconstruction on early continence after robot-assisted laparoscopic radical prostatectomy: results of a prospective parallel group trial. Eur Urol. 2010;58(1):84–9.
64. Menon M, Muhletaler F, Campos M, Peabody JO. Assessment of early continence after reconstruction of the periprostatic tissues in patients undergoing computer assisted (robotic) prostatectomy: results of a 2 group parallel randomized controlled trial. J Urol. 2008;180(3):1018–23.
65. Sammon JD, Muhletaler F, Peabody JO, Diaz-Insua M, Satyanaryana R, Menon M. Long-term functional urinary outcomes comparing single- vs double-layer urethrovesical anastomosis: two-year follow-up of a two-group parallel randomized controlled trial. Urology. 2010;76(5):1102–7.
66. Hurtes X, Roupret M, Vaessen C, Pereira H, Faivre d'Arcier B, Cormier L, et al. Anterior suspension combined with posterior reconstruction during robot-assisted laparoscopic prostatectomy improves early return of urinary continence: a prospective randomized multicentre trial. BJU Int. 2012;110(6):875–83.
67. Tewari A, Jhaveri J, Rao S, Yadav R, Bartsch G, Te A, et al. Total reconstruction of the vesicourethral junction. BJU Int. 2008;101(7):871–7.

Chapter 2
Preoperative Assessment and Intervention: Optimizing Outcomes for Early Return of Urinary Continence

Fouad Aoun, Simone Albisinni, Ksenija Limani, and Roland van Velthoven

Introduction

The introduction of robotic surgery for the treatment of prostate cancer has allowed for the collection of more accurate anatomical information on adjacent prostatic structures and has facilitated innovative techniques aimed at enhancing postoperative functional results without compromising oncological prognosis. However, despite improved surgical technique and expertise, urinary incontinence still occurs in the early postoperative setting with an incidence varying between 6 and 20 % [1, 2]. Spontaneous recovery of urinary incontinence is generally to be expected within 3–24 months after surgery but is variable among patients even when a standard approach is applied by the same surgeon [3]. These findings highlight the importance of underlying preoperative factors influencing continence recovery and the timing of recovery. Preoperative evaluation of these factors can provide precious information about postoperative continence. This may help surgeons to individually tailor their approach in accordance with tumor- and patient-related factors to accelerate continence recovery and give patients better preoperative counseling and more legitimate expectations. Herein, we analyzed significant preoperative factors and their assessment techniques that are predictors of early return of urinary continence. Preoperative intervention for modifiable factors and individualized treatment based on preoperative factors in order to achieve early urinary continence were also summarized.

F. Aoun, M.D., M.Sc. (✉)
Department of Urology, Institut Jules Bordet, Brussels, Belgium

Saint Joseph University, Hotel Dieu de France, Beirut, Lebanon
e-mail: fouad.aoun@bordet.be

S. Albisinni, M.D. • K. Limani, M.D. • R. van Velthoven, M.D., Ph.D.
Department of Urology, Institut Jules Bordet, Brussels, Belgium

© Springer International Publishing Switzerland 2016
S. Razdan (ed.), *Urinary Continence and Sexual Function After Robotic Radical Prostatectomy*, DOI 10.1007/978-3-319-39448-0_2

Preoperative Factors Predictive of Continence Recovery After Radical Prostatectomy

Several patient- and tumor-related preoperative predictors of early return of urinary continence following radical prostatectomy have been evaluated in various publications. Patient's age at surgery is the most reported preoperative nonmodifiable factor compromising the continence status. In a population-based longitudinal cohort study, men aged <60 years were significantly less likely to have postoperative incontinence than older men [4]. Men aged 75–79 years experienced the highest level of incontinence compared to younger patients. In a prospective study, Talcott et al. reported that the continence rate at 12 months was 91 % among patients aged <65 years and 85 % among those aged ≥65 years at surgery [5]. In a recent study, a significant correlation between age and immediate continence after catheter removal was detected [6]. Similarly, Compodonico et al. showed that younger age <65 years was independently associated with immediate continence (OR = 2.63, 95 % CI 1.13–5.88, $p = 0.02$) on multivariate logistic analysis [7]. However, in other studies, the age at surgery had no significant effect on early return of urinary continence but these series either included few elderly patients or observed low rates of incontinence rendering identification of significant risk factors unlikely [8, 9]. Performance status in the preoperative setting was also demonstrated to correlate with early achievement of continence. A favorable Eastern Cooperation Oncology Group (ECOG) of 0 performance score was found as an independent predictor factor for immediate continence in the study of Hatiboglu et al. [6]. Preoperative potency represents also a positive predictor factor of early return of urinary continence in patients treated with bilateral nerve sparing radical prostatectomy. Severe preoperative erectile dysfunction had been demonstrated to be associated with less nerve sparing procedure and thus, worse urinary continence outcome [6, 10, 11]. In addition, several studies have suggested that body mass index (BMI) and baseline physical activity play an important role in regaining postprostatectomy continence levels. Men who were not obese and were active were 26 % less likely to be incontinent than men who were obese and inactive in a study published by Wolin et al. [12]. However, it seems that BMI is not a prognostic factor for immediate continence as evidenced in the study of Hatiboglu et al. [6]. In the CaPSURE national disease registry of men with prostate cancer, preoperative prostate volume was a predictor of recovery of urinary function after radical prostatectomy. Men with prostate volume greater than 50 cc had lower rates of continence, as assessed by urinary function scores 6 months and 1 year after radical prostatectomy, but scores equalized across all volume ranges by 2 years after radical prostatectomy. The individual domains most significantly affected were urinary control, urine leakage, frequency and urine leakage during sexual activity [13]. A potential reason could be subclinical bladder dysfunction related to benign prostatic hyperplasia that is unmasked by surgery. In fact, bladder dysfunction was also demonstrated as a rare cause of incontinence in some patients [14]. Moreover, preoperative bladder dysfunction mainly overactive bladder is a common problem encountered in 40–50 % of patients [15, 16].

These dysfunctions are, in the majority of cases, compensated and/or subclinical. They tend to deteriorate after surgery and may exacerbate incontinence associated with sphincteric insufficiency [17]. Higher preoperative maximal urethral closure pressure (MUCP) was demonstrated in men regaining continence at 6 months post-operatively compared with incontinent patients and poor preoperative MUCP was independently correlated with persistent incontinence postoperatively [18]. Functional urethral length is another urodynamic parameter that significantly decreases after radical prostatectomy [19]. However, its role as a diagnostic preoperative tool is controversial and more well-designed studies are needed to support its use as a preoperative predictor of postoperative risk of urinary incontinence. Similarly, detrusor function and pressure flow parameters were not predictors of early regain of continence but further prospective diagnostic accuracy studies are still needed to elucidate the role of these studies in the preoperative period [18]. Finally, baseline incontinence is understandably associated with higher rates of incontinence postoperatively [20].

Effect of Anatomical Interindividual Variations on Early Return of Urinary Continence

The preprostatectomy surgical anatomy of the male pelvic floor and perineal anatomy is complex and varies substantially. The external urethral sphincter is a complex structure surrounding the membranous urethra from the apex of the prostate to the penile bulb, in the shape of an inverted horseshoe. It is in close anatomic and functional relationship to the pelvic floor, and its fragile innervation is in close association to the prostate apex. Thus, the shape and size of the prostate can significantly modify the anatomy of the NVB and the urethral sphincter [21, 22]. Muscle fibers and/or nerve supply injury during dissection may result in urethral sphincter insufficiency and cause postoperative urinary incontinence. Understandably, the shape of the prostate at the apex influences the length of the membranous urethra [23]. The external urethral sphincter could in some cases be surrounded by the apex circumferentially making its preservation difficult particularly if the tumor is located at the apex. A long urethral stump is a well-known predictor factor of postoperative immediate continence [24, 25]. Therefore, a preoperative long membranous urethral length and the absence of overlapping between the prostatic apex and the membranous urethra should correlate with higher rates of recovery of urinary continence after radical prostatectomy. Interestingly, Paparel et al. confirmed this hypothesis by demonstrating that time to recovery of urinary incontinence was strongly associated with preoperative membranous urethral length [26]. In fact, a postoperative length >13 mm guaranty immediate continence whereas 70 % of patients had immediate continence when membranous urethral length <13 mm. Lee et al. demonstrated that a prostatic apex overlapping the membranous urethra had a higher risk of excessive shortening of the urethra after the intervention and therefore accounting for a delay in return of urinary continence [27]. A Korean study described the same findings [23]; patients without an anterior or posterior overlying apical pattern had greater chance of early return of continence and higher rates of continence at 1 year of follow-up. However, Mendoza et al. did not find a cutoff value for urethral length [28]. The length of the prostate was also evoked as another anatomical factor that influences urinary recovery after the intervention. Arguably, longer prostates are associated with a greater damage to the NVBs; however, there are some data showing no significant correlation between the prostate length and the early return to continence in the postoperative period [23, 26]. Levator ani thickness at the height of apical dissection, urethral volume, recto-urethralis muscles, puboprostatic ligaments, outer and inner levator distance had been also studied but results are contradictory [18]. All these anatomical variations can be detected and measured in the preoperative period and analyzed and compared to the postoperative setting. Sphincter electromyography and perfusion sphincterometry did not prove their utility for preoperative evaluation of urethral sphincter function for patients awaiting radical prostatectomy [29, 30]. This stems mainly from the normal sphincter function in the majority of patients. Comparison between preoperative and postoperative patterns failed to categorize a subgroup of patients at increased risk for delayed return of continence [31, 32]. On the other hand, membranous urethral length is best assessed by endorectal MRI and several studies investigated its role in augmenting the prediction of continence recovery. Coakley et al. examined 211 patients by MRI before radical prostatectomy and demonstrated the rapid return of urinary continence after the procedure [33]. Von Bodman et al. obtained the same results in a retrospective series of 600 patients [34]. Lim et al. suggested, in their studies, that assessing apical shape on a preoperative mid-sagittal MRI was as much important as measuring the urethral length in predicting early return to continence [23]. However, the absence of a standardized method for measuring anatomical interindividual variability, the retrospective design of the studies, and the low predictive accuracy of these tests limit their reproducibility and their routine use in everyday practice.

The Value of Preoperative Intervention Aimed to Enhance Early Return of Urinary Continence Following Radical Prostatectomy

Individualization of treatment to reduce therapy-associated early and late functional morbidity is the current trend in cancer surgery. The extent of dissection should be adapted according to patient- and tumor-related factors. Distinguishing patients into different subgroups based on their preoperative risk factors for postoperative delayed recovery of incontinence is an emerging concept in the surgical management of prostate cancer [35]. Patients with idiopathic detrusor overactivity including those with abnormally low bladder compliance are at increased risk for postoperative incontinence. Good urodynamic assessment of these patients and preoperative or simultaneous use of botulinum toxin could decrease incontinence after radical prostatectomy as demonstrated in small series (Abdulhak A, Abst ICS). The effect of botulinum toxin on prostate cancer cells remains to be elucidated [36]. Patients experiencing preoperative urinary incontinence should be informed of their highest risk of incontinence after the intervention. Physical activity and weight loss could play a role in reducing the time to regain continence after radical prostatectomy and are encouraged [12]. Accurate tumor localization is also of paramount importance in tailoring management of prostate cancer. Higher clinical stage, PSA levels, and preoperative Gleason score were shown to predict worse urinary continence outcome [37]. However, tumor stage, PSA, and D'Amico risk groups were not found to be significant predictors of early return of continence in recent series [6]. Understandably, increased tumor aggressiveness is associated with a higher rate of positive surgical margins and biochemical recurrence that might be treated with postoperative radiation therapy with a substantial negative impact on urinary continence outcomes. Morphological alterations in periprostatic tissues due to changes in cancer microenvironment in aggressive tumor need to be confirmed. A short membranous urethral length with an overlapping prostatic apex and an aggressive tumor located at the apex expose the patient to higher risk of positive surgical margins and/or persistent urinary incontinence [38, 39]. Robotic approach could facilitate apical dissection in the confined space particularly if posterior pubic tuberosity is prominent allowing better visualization and access to the limits of dissection but in the absence of oncologic and functional data, many surgeons prefer to offer radiation therapy for these patients to avoid the higher risk of persistent urinary incontinence [40, 41]. Patients with weak pelvic floor muscles or preoperative sphincteric insufficiency could be offered pelvic floor muscle training (PFMT). However, the clinical utility of preoperative PFMT which has been demonstrated for the management of female stress urinary incontinence [42] is more contradictory in men. The principle is based on the assumption that increasing pelvic muscle tone may improve its support to pelvic structures during moments of involuntary increase in intra-abdominal pressure, thus reducing urinary leaking during efforts. In order to ameliorate continence recovery after RALP, investigators have tested the impact of PFMT before the surgical operation. Indeed, it may be thought that a muscular preparation of the pelvic floor prior to the surgical trauma can potentially be beneficial in order to accelerate and improve continence outcomes. Generally, patients start the training 2–4 weeks before surgery and then continue after postoperative catheter retrieval. In addition, the technique may be guided by electromyographic biofeedback or by a physiotherapist; exercise schedule is variable, usually including one weekly encounter with the physiotherapist and daily home contraction exercises. Although theoretically effective in "training" the pelvic floor, multiple RCTs exploring preoperative PFMT have reported variable and contrasting results, and its true clinical impact has yet been elucidated. In summary, current data do not support the use of preoperative PFMT, which does not seem to improve continence outcomes after prostatectomy, neither on the short nor on the long term [43]. However, given the noninvasiveness of PFMT and the high percentage of patient satisfaction, some experts still recommend its use before surgery, particularly in patients at risk but its true impact on quality of life and time to continence requires further investigation.

Conclusion

In the future, the variability in time to regain continence could be predicted in the preoperative setting and thus helps in the patient decision making. Urologist should be aware of the possibilities of these diagnostic tools. A combination of preoperative MRI and urethral pressure profilometry measurements could be used to predict early return of continence. However, more and larger prospective studies with validated and standardized tools are needed to determine the exact role, the clinical utility, and the cost effectiveness of these techniques preoperatively. The next step could be a more individualized approach based on preoperative patient- and tumor-related factors. Tailoring surgery according to these factors could reduce urinary functional complications without compromising oncological outcomes.

References

1. Coughlin G, Palmer KJ, Shah K, Patel VR. Robotic-assisted radical prostatectomy: functional outcomes. Arch Esp Urol. 2007;60(4):408–18.
2. Mottrie A, Van Migem P, De Naeyer G, Schatteman P, Carpentier P, Fonteyne E. Robot-assisted laparoscopic radical prostatectomy: oncologic and functional results of 184 cases. Eur Urol. 2007;52(3):746–50. doi:10.1016/j.eururo.2007.02.029.
3. Menon M, Shrivastava A, Kaul S, Badani KK, Fumo M, Bhandari M, et al. Vattikuti Institute prostatectomy: contemporary technique and analysis of results. Eur Urol. 2007;51(3):648–57. doi:10.1016/j.eururo.2006.10.055. discussion 657-648.
4. Stanford JL, Feng Z, Hamilton AS, Gilliland FD, Stephenson RA, Eley JW, et al. Urinary and sexual function after radical prostatectomy for clinically localized prostate cancer: the Prostate Cancer Outcomes Study. JAMA. 2000;283(3):354–60.
5. Talcott JA, Rieker P, Clark JA, Propert KJ, Weeks JC, Beard CJ, et al. Patient-reported symptoms after primary therapy for early prostate cancer: results of a prospective cohort study. J Clin Oncol. 1998;16(1):275–83.
6. Hatiboglu G, Teber D, Tichy D, Pahernik S, Hadaschik B, Nyarangi-Dix J, et al. Predictive factors for immediate continence after radical prostatectomy. World J Urol. 2015. doi:10.1007/s00345-015-1594-4.
7. Campodonico F, Manuputty EE, Campora S, Puntoni M, Maffezzini M. Age is predictive of immediate postoperative urinary continence after radical retropubic prostatectomy. Urol Int. 2014;92(3):276–81. doi:10.1159/000353414.
8. Geary ES, Dendinger TE, Freiha FS, Stamey TA. Incontinence and vesical neck strictures following radical retropubic prostatectomy. Urology. 1995;45(6):1000–6.
9. Eastham JA, Kattan MW, Rogers E, Goad JR, Ohori M, Boone TB, et al. Risk factors for urinary incontinence after radical prostatectomy. J Urol. 1996;156(5):1707–13.
10. Sammon JD, Sharma P, Trinh QD, Ghani KR, Sukumar S, Menon M. Predictors of immediate continence following robot-assisted radical prostatectomy. J Endourol. 2013;27(4):442–6. doi:10.1089/end.2012.0312.
11. Srivastava A, Chopra S, Pham A, Sooriakumaran P, Durand M, Chughtai B, et al. Effect of a risk-stratified grade of nerve-sparing technique on early return of continence after robot-assisted laparoscopic radical prostatectomy. Eur Urol. 2013;63(3):438–44. doi:10.1016/j.eururo.2012.07.009.
12. Wolin KY, Luly J, Sutcliffe S, Andriole GL, Kibel AS. Risk of urinary incontinence following prostatectomy: the role of physical activity and obesity. J Urol. 2010;183(2):629–33. doi:10.1016/j.juro.2009.09.082.

13. Konety BR, Sadetsky N, Carroll PR, Ca PI. Recovery of urinary continence following radical prostatectomy: the impact of prostate volume—analysis of data from the CaPSURE Database. J Urol. 2007;177(4):1423–5. doi:10.1016/j.juro.2006.11.089. discussion 1425-1426.
14. Groutz A, Blaivas JG, Chaikin DC, Weiss JP, Verhaaren M. The pathophysiology of post-radical prostatectomy incontinence: a clinical and video urodynamic study. J Urol. 2000;163(6): 1767–70.
15. Giannantoni A, Mearini E, Di Stasi SM, Mearini L, Bini V, Pizzirusso G, et al. Assessment of bladder and urethral sphincter function before and after radical retropubic prostatectomy. J Urol. 2004;171(4):1563–6. doi:10.1097/01.ju.0000118957.24390.66.
16. Song C, Lee J, Hong JH, Choo MS, Kim CS, Ahn H. Urodynamic interpretation of changing bladder function and voiding pattern after radical prostatectomy: a long-term follow-up. BJU Int. 2010;106(5):681–6. doi:10.1111/j.1464-410X.2009.09189.x.
17. Hammerer P, Huland H. Urodynamic evaluation of changes in urinary control after radical retropubic prostatectomy. J Urol. 1997;157(1):233–6.
18. Dubbelman YD, Groen J, Wildhagen MF, Rikken B, Bosch JL. Urodynamic quantification of decrease in sphincter function after radical prostatectomy: relation to postoperative continence status and the effect of intensive pelvic floor muscle exercises. NeurourolUrodyn. 2012;31(5):646–51. doi:10.1002/nau.21243.
19. Pfister C, Cappele O, Dunet F, Bugel H, Grise P. Assessment of the intrinsic urethral sphincter component function in postprostatectomy urinary incontinence. NeurourolUrodyn. 2002; 21(3):194–7.
20. Moore KN, Truong V, Estey E, Voaklander DC. Urinary incontinence after radical prostatectomy: can men at risk be identified preoperatively? J Wound Ostomy Continence Nurs. 2007;34(3):270–9. doi:10.1097/01.WON.0000270821.91694.56. quiz 280-271.
21. Sipal T, Tuglu D, Yilmaz E, Atasoy P, Batislam E. Continence recovery time after radical prostatectomy: implication of prostatic apical tumor. Minerva Urol Nefrol. 2013;65(3): 197–203.
22. Walz J, Burnett AL, Costello AJ, Eastham JA, Graefen M, Guillonneau B, et al. A critical analysis of the current knowledge of surgical anatomy related to optimization of cancer control and preservation of continence and erection in candidates for radical prostatectomy. Eur Urol. 2010;57(2):179–92. doi:10.1016/j.eururo.2009.11.009.
23. Lim TJ, Lee JH, Lim JW, Moon SK, Jeon SH, Chang SG. Preoperative factors predictive of continence recovery after radical retropubic prostatectomy. Korean J Urol. 2012;53(8):524–30. doi:10.4111/kju.2012.53.8.524.
24. Hamada A, Razdan S, Etafy MH, Fagin R, Razdan S. Early return of continence in patients undergoing robot-assisted laparoscopic prostatectomy using modified maximal urethral length preservation technique. J Endourol. 2014;28(8):930–8. doi:10.1089/end.2013.0794.
25. Borin JF, Skarecky DW, Narula N, Ahlering TE. Impact of urethral stump length on continence and positive surgical margins in robot-assisted laparoscopic prostatectomy. Urology. 2007;70(1):173–7. doi:10.1016/j.urology.2007.03.050.
26. Paparel P, Akin O, Sandhu JS, Otero JR, Serio AM, Scardino PT, et al. Recovery of urinary continence after radical prostatectomy: association with urethral length and urethral fibrosis measured by preoperative and postoperative endorectal magnetic resonance imaging. Eur Urol. 2009;55(3):629–37. doi:10.1016/j.eururo.2008.08.057.
27. Lee SE, Byun SS, Lee HJ, Song SH, Chang IH, Kim YJ, et al. Impact of variations in prostatic apex shape on early recovery of urinary continence after radical retropubic prostatectomy. Urology. 2006;68(1):137–41. doi:10.1016/j.urology.2006.01.021.
28. Mendoza PJ, Stern JM, Li AY, Jaffe W, Kovell R, Nguyen M, et al. Pelvic anatomy on preoperative magnetic resonance imaging can predict early continence after robot-assisted radical prostatectomy. J Endourol. 2011;25(1):51–5. doi:10.1089/end.2010.0184.
29. Desautel MG, Kapoor R, Badlani GH. Sphincteric incontinence: the primary cause of post-prostatectomy incontinence in patients with prostate cancer. NeurourolUrodyn. 1997;16(3):153–60.
30. Ficazzola MA, Nitti VW. The etiology of post-radical prostatectomy incontinence and correlation of symptoms with urodynamic findings. J Urol. 1998;160(4):1317–20.

31. Gudziak MR, McGuire EJ, Gormley EA. Urodynamic assessment of urethral sphincter function in post-prostatectomy incontinence. J Urol. 1996;156(3):1131–4. discussion 1134-1135.
32. Winters JC, Appell RA, Rackley RR. Urodynamic findings in postprostatectomy incontinence. NeurourolUrodyn. 1998;17(5):493–8.
33. Coakley FV, Eberhardt S, Kattan MW, Wei DC, Scardino PT, Hricak H. Urinary continence after radical retropubic prostatectomy: relationship with membranous urethral length on pre-operative endorectal magnetic resonance imaging. J Urol. 2002;168(3):1032–5. doi:10.1097/01.ju.0000025881.75827.a5.
34. von Bodman C, Matsushita K, Savage C, Matikainen MP, Eastham JA, Scardino PT, et al. Recovery of urinary function after radical prostatectomy: predictors of urinary function on preoperative prostate magnetic resonance imaging. J Urol. 2012;187(3):945–50. doi:10.1016/j.juro.2011.10.143.
35. Jeong SJ, Yeon JS, Lee JK, Cha WH, Jeong JW, Lee BK, et al. Development and validation of nomograms to predict the recovery of urinary continence after radical prostatectomy: comparisons between immediate, early, and late continence. World J Urol. 2014;32(2):437–44. doi:10.1007/s00345-013-1127-y.
36. Karsenty G, Rocha J, Chevalier S, Scarlata E, Andrieu C, Zouanat FZ, et al. Botulinum toxin type A inhibits the growth of LNCaP human prostate cancer cells in vitro and in vivo. Prostate. 2009;69(11):1143–50. doi:10.1002/pros.20958.
37. Egawa S, Minei S, Iwamura M, Uchida T, Koshiba K. Urinary continence following radical prostatectomy. Jpn J Clin Oncol. 1997;27(2):71–5.
38. Preston MA, Blute ML. Positive surgical margins after radical prostatectomy: does it matter? Eur Urol. 2014;65(2):314–5. doi:10.1016/j.eururo.2013.08.037.
39. Weidner N, Carroll PR, Flax J, Blumenfeld W, Folkman J. Tumor angiogenesis correlates with metastasis in invasive prostate carcinoma. Am J Pathol. 1993;143(2):401–9.
40. Kim SC, Song C, Kim W, Kang T, Park J, Jeong IG, et al. Factors determining functional outcomes after radical prostatectomy: robot-assisted versus retropubic. Eur Urol. 2011;60(3):413–9. doi:10.1016/j.eururo.2011.05.011.
41. Son SJ, Lee SC, Jeong CW, Jeong SJ, Byun SS, Lee SE. Comparison of continence recovery between robot-assisted laparoscopic prostatectomy and open radical retropubic prostatectomy: a single surgeon experience. Korean J Urol. 2013;54(9):598–602. doi:10.4111/kju.2013.54.9.598.
42. Lucas MG, Bosch RJ, Burkhard FC, Cruz F, Madden TB, Nambiar AK, Neisius A, de Ridder DJ, Tubaro A, Turner WH, Pickard RS, European Association of U. EAU guidelines on assessment and nonsurgical management of urinary incontinence. Eur Urol. 2012;62(6):1130–42. doi:10.1016/j.eururo.2012.08.047.
43. Wang W, Huang QM, Liu FP, Mao QQ. Effectiveness of preoperative pelvic floor muscle training for urinary incontinence after radical prostatectomy: a meta-analysis. BMC Urol. 2014;14:99. doi:10.1186/1471-2490-14-99.

Chapter 3
Preoperative Assessment and Intervention: Optimizing Outcomes for Early Return of Erectile Function

Weil R. Lai and Raju Thomas

Introduction

Erectile dysfunction (ED) is one of the most common treatment-related side effects following a radical prostatectomy for prostate cancer. ED is defined as "the persistent inability to attain and maintain an erection sufficient to permit satisfactory sexual performance" [1]. To the authors' best knowledge, while there have been no published studies evaluating the preoperative optimization of patients to increase in erectile function return after radical prostatectomy, there have been numerous studies done to evaluate the interventions in modifiable risk factors to improve erectile function. This chapter aims to review such studies and discuss potential pathways to optimize patients preoperatively for erectile function recovery after radical prostatectomy.

Epidemiology

Many patients already have underlying ED prior to the diagnosis of prostate cancer. ED is diagnosed worldwide and not unique to any one specific medical condition. One of the first longitudinal studies evaluating erectile function was the Massachusetts Male Aging Study (MMAS) [2]. In this study, a cohort of noninstitutionalized men, ages 40–70 and living in the Greater Boston area, were initially surveyed between 1987 and 1989, and then resurveyed between 1995 and 1997. MMAS showed that over the two surveys, the prevalence of ED increased as follows: complete ED from 5.1 to 15 %, moderate ED from 17 to 34 %, and mild ED remaining constant around 17 % [2]. In the National Health and Social Life Survey (NHSLS), which surveyed

W.R. Lai, M.D. • R. Thomas, M.D., F.A.C.S., M.H.A. (✉)
Department of Urology, Tulane University School of Medicine,
1430 Tulane Ave., SL-42, New Orleans, LA 70112, USA
e-mail: rthomas@tulane.edu

© Springer International Publishing Switzerland 2016
S. Razdan (ed.), *Urinary Continence and Sexual Function After Robotic Radical Prostatectomy*, DOI 10.1007/978-3-319-39448-0_3

men between 18 and 59 years of age in the United States, the prevalence of ED increased with age: 7 % for ages 18–29, 9 % for ages 30–39, 11 % for ages 40–49, and 18 % for ages 50–59 [3]. This finding is supported in a comprehensive literature review by Lewis et al. [4]. In their analysis of 59 studies reporting the prevalence of ED, these authors showed that the worldwide prevalence for ED increased with age as follows: 1–10 % below age 40, 2–15 % for ages 40–49, 6–55 % for ages 50–59, 20–40 % for ages 60–69, and 50–100 % for ages 70–80s.

Evaluation of ED

The evaluation of ED should include a detailed medical and sexual history. Medical history may identify comorbidities and medications associated with ED. Sexual history can be supplemented with validated patient self-reported questionnaires. The International Index for Erectile Function (IIEF) is a commonly used questionnaire [5], consisting of 15 questions covering the following five domains: erectile function, orgasmic function, sexual desire, intercourse satisfaction, and overall satisfaction. For the purpose of diagnosing the presence and severity of ED, an abbreviated version of only five questions (IIEF-5) has been developed and used commonly in the clinical and research settings [6]. Such surveys have been used in clinical trials to quantify the degree of treatment response to ED interventions [7]. Other published instruments in the assessment of ED include the Brief Male Sexual Function Inventory [8], Center for Marital and Sexual Health Sexual Functioning Questionnaire [9], Changes in Sexual Functioning Questionnaire [10], Erectile Dysfunction Inventory of Treatment Satisfaction [11], Male Sexual Health Questionnaire [12], and Sexual Experience Questionnaire [13].

As there may be multiple etiologies/contributors of ED, physical examination should include components from the cardiovascular (e.g., signs of hypertension), endocrine (e.g., signs of hypogonadism), neurologic, and genitourinary systems (e.g., penile plaques) [14]. Laboratory testing includes assessment of glycemic control (e.g., fasting glucose or HgbA1c), lipid profile, and serum testosterone.

Classification of ED

ED was historically thought to be mostly psychogenic in etiology. In 1965, Masters and Johnson estimated that psychogenic ED affected approximately 90 % of impotent men [15]. With the improved understanding of erection physiology, many studies have proposed classification schemes for the etiology of ED. The classification recommended by the International Society of Impotence Research in 1999 [16] divides ED into organic and psychogenic etiologies. Organic etiologies can be subdivided into vasculogenic, neurogenic, anatomic, endocrinologic, medication, and trauma etiologies. Psychogenic etiologies can be subdivided into generalized and situational etiologies (Fig. 3.1).

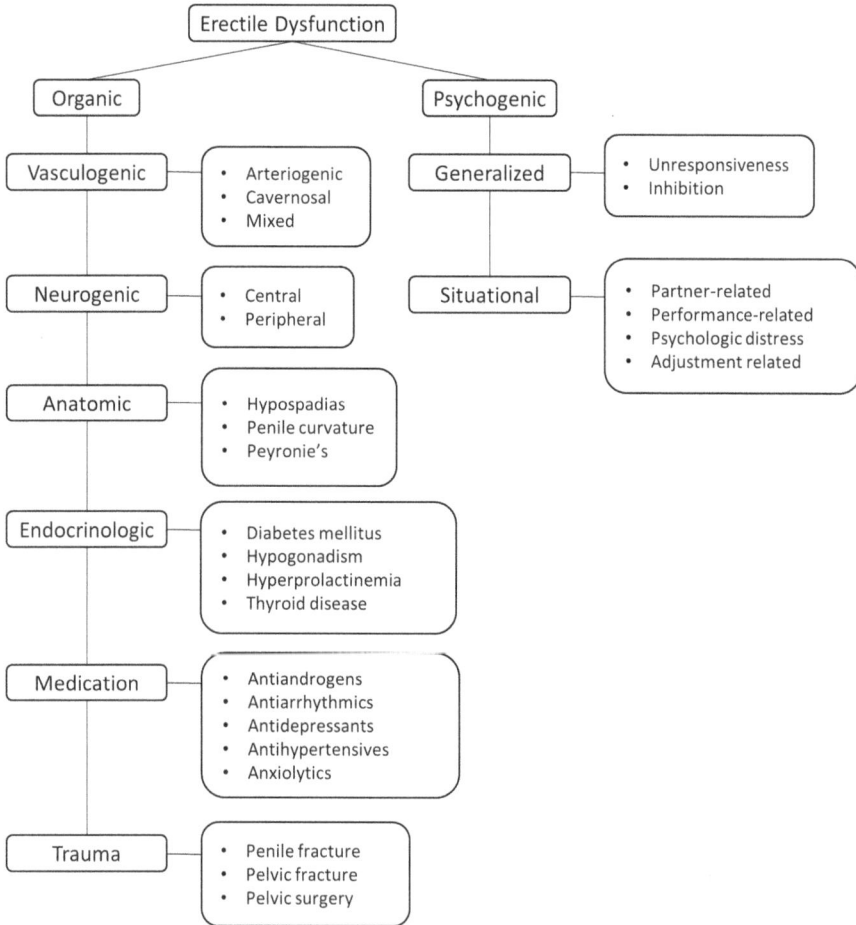

Fig. 3.1 Classifications of erectile dysfunction

Risk Factors

ED-related risk factors have been well characterized in population studies. In a multivariate analysis of the 2001–2002 National Health and Nutrition Examination Survey (comprising of data from 2126 adult males), ED was significantly and independently associated with diabetes mellitus, lower attained education, and lack of physical activity [17]. A different group of authors analyzing the same survey reported obstructive urinary symptoms, hypertension with selected antihypertensive therapy, and selected antidepressant therapy as additional risk factors that are independently and statistically associated with the increased risk of ED [18]. Other comorbidities (e.g., obesity, cigarette smoking, alcohol abuse, recreational drug use, dyslipidemia, hypogonadism) are also associated with ED [14]. Classes of medications associated with ED include antiandrogens, antihypertensives (e.g., thiazides, beta-blockers, calcium channel blockers), antiarrhythmics (e.g., digoxin, amiodarone, disopyramide, HMG-CoA reductase inhibitors), and psychotropic drugs (e.g., tricyclic antidepressants, selective serotonin reuptake inhibitors, phenothiazines, butyrophenones) [14].

Physical Activity Studies

As ED can be an early marker of cardiovascular disease [19], the interventions to improve cardiovascular health have been evaluated, in multiple studies, for demonstrated benefit in erectile function. Lifestyle modifications such as increased physical activity have been shown to ameliorate ED.

In a meta-analysis evaluating the relationship between physical activity and ED [20], seven cross-sectional studies were selected for the analysis. The studies defined ED either by IIEF or by the patient's ability "to get and keep an erection adequate for satisfactory intercourse." The studies included patients from Brazil, Turkey, Italy, Japan, Malaysia, Belgium, Korea, and Singapore. Moderate and high physical activities were found to be significantly associated with a lower risk of ED (odds ratios of 0.63 and 0.42, respectively).

In a randomized controlled trial (RCT) of 43 hypertensive men with ED [21], the participants were randomized into exercise and control groups. The exercise group was enrolled in an 8-week training program with a bicycle ergometer. The control group remained sedentary during the study period. To reduce risk of competing comorbidities, the study selected men with few comorbidities (e.g., those with obesity, diabetes, tobacco use, alcohol abuse, and other systemic diseases were excluded). Mean age was 62.1 and 64 for the exercise and control groups, respectively. In addition to showing significant reduction in systolic and diastolic blood pressure and reduction in serum C-reactive protein in the exercise group, the study also found reduced ED, from a mean IIEF of 11.5 to 15.1 ($p < 0.05$).

In a prospective cohort study of 50 patients with arterial ED, the patients underwent 150 min of moderate intensity aerobic activity per week and were counseled to abide by the Mediterranean diet [22]. Mean age was 57.3 years. These 50 patients were compared to 20 additional control patients who observed only the principles of the Mediterranean diet. After 3 months, the intervention group showed significant improvement in the peak systolic velocity, acceleration time, IIEF-5 (from 11 to 16.5), BMI, total cholesterol, HDL cholesterol, triglycerides, systolic blood pressure, and diastolic blood pressure. The interventional group also showed significant decrease in circulating endothelial progenitor cells and decreased percentage of circulating endothelial microparticles, which represent a reduction in endothelial repair and endothelial apoptosis.

In another 60-patient RCT [23], males 40–60 years of age affected by ED and considered inactive (defined as less than 2 h of exercise per week) were randomized to receive phosphodiesterase-5 inhibitors (PDE-5i) alone (control) or PDE-5i plus regular, aerobic physical activity (i.e., an exercise regimen of at least 3 h per week). After 3 months, IIEF restoration of erectile function occurred in 77.8 % of the physical activity group and 39.3 % of the controls. On multivariate logistic regression analysis, physical activity was the only independent variable for normal erection ($p=0.01$), higher sexual satisfaction ($p=0.022$), and normal total IIEF score ($p=0.023$). As a measure of validity, the physical activity group did exercise a mean of 3.4 h per week (compared to 0.45 h per week for the controls). This study suggested that adding physical activity to PDE-5i therapy might further improve erectile function.

Weight Loss Studies

Obesity has been shown in multiple epidemiologic studies to be associated with an increased risk of ED. In the Health Professionals Follow-up Study, which consisted of 31,742 male health care professionals who responded to the questionnaires over a 14-year period, those with obesity (defined in the study as a body mass index— BMI—greater than 28.7 kg/m^2 based on cutoff established for the fifth quintile of the study population) had a 30 % increased risk for ED compared to their nonobese counterparts (BMI less than 23.2 kg/m^2) [24]. These findings were also seen in the MMAS and other similar cross-sectional studies. The Androx Vienna study evaluated blue-collar workers ages 45–60 years with questionnaires, health exams, and blood samples [25]. Analysis of the Androx Vienna study group showed that an increase of BMI by 1 kg/m^2 reduced IIEF-5 by 0.141, independent of age. In multiple logistic regression analyses, this study also showed an increase in ED risk by 7.6 % per kg/m^2 of BMI and 8.2 % per year of age.

To evaluate the effect of caloric restriction on sexual function, a prospective cohort study in Australia recruited obese men (BMI greater or equal to 30 kg/m^2) into a weight loss program [26]. In the intervention group ($n=44$; 19 were diabetic), the men consumed low-calorie meal replacements for breakfast and lunch and/or dinner. The control group ($n=24$; none were diabetic) remained on their usual diet during the study. After 8 weeks on the low-calorie diet, diabetic and nondiabetic men in the interventional group increased IIEF-5 scores significantly by 2.1 (i.e., from 8.1 to 10.2) and 2.2 (i.e., from 17.8 to 20), respectively. Sexual Desire Inventory scores increased significantly by 10.4 (i.e., from 44.1 to 54.5) and 9.1 (i.e., from 71.2 to 80.3), respectively. The interventional group lost, on average, 10 % of their weight and demonstrated improved insulin sensitivity index. The control group showed no change over the duration of the study.

In a separate prospective study from the same group in Australia [27], 31 obese men with well-controlled Type 2 diabetes mellitus were randomized to a low-caloric diet ($n=19$) or a high-protein, low-fat diet ($n=12$). Those on the low-caloric diet remained on this diet for 8 weeks and then were switched to the high-protein, low-fat diet. Both groups were followed for 52 weeks. At 8 weeks, the low-calorie and high-protein groups increased IIEF-5 by 2.2 and 2.8, respectively. At 52 weeks, IIEF-5 increased by 6.8 and 6.7, respectively. Weight loss percentage at 52 weeks was 8.5 and 8.2 %, respectively. For both diets (at 8 weeks), improvements were also seen in sex hormone binding globulin, International Prostate Symptom Score (IPSS), sE-selectin, glucose, and low-density lipoprotein. At 52 weeks, further improvements were also seen in IPSS, sE-selectin, triglycerides, and low-density lipoprotein.

A RCT in Singapore randomized 48 obese Asian men (defined as BMI greater than or equal to 27.5 kg/m^2) to receive either a conventional reduced fat diet or a low caloric diet [28]. Those on the low caloric diet (which was 400 kcal/day lower than the conventional diet) were switched to the conventional diet at 12 weeks. Both groups were advised to perform moderate-intensity exercise. At 12 weeks, the low caloric diet group lost more weight than the conventional diet group (−4.2 versus −2.5 kg, respectively). At 40 weeks, the degree of weight loss was maintained. The proportion of ED at baseline was similar between the two groups (75 % versus 83.3 %). Both groups significantly improved IIEF-5 at 12 weeks (from 17.2 to 20.5 and 17.9 to 20.4, respectively) and maintained the improvement at 40 weeks. Improvement in IIEF-5 was significantly associated with waist circumference reduction, increase in total testosterone, and endothelial function (measured via the Reactive Hyperemia Index).

Weight loss achieved secondary to the effects of bariatric surgery also demonstrated improvements in erectile function. A RCT from Brazil studied 20 patients with morbid obesity for 2 years [29]. Ten underwent Roux-en-Y gastric bypass at 4 months after having undergone a program consisting of daily physical activity and nutritional education for a low energy diet. The remaining 10 patients (controls) did not receive the intensive program. The investigators excluded those with tobacco/alcohol abuse and those taking PDE-5i, antihypertensives, diabetic medications, or statins. At 4 months, the intervention group dropped its mean BMI significantly from 55.7 to 43.1; IIEF-5 and hormonal parameters were unchanged. At 2 years, the intervention group dropped its mean BMI further to 31; IIEF-5 increased significantly from 19.7 to 23. Total and free testosterone also increased significantly, while prolactin decreased significantly. In comparison, the control group showed no changes at 4 months and at 2 years. Of note, the mean PSAs at baseline were 0.7 and 0.6 ng/mL for the intervention and control groups, respectively.

In a prospective cohort series of 97 men who underwent gastric bypass for morbid obesity [30], the authors assessed sexual function pre- and postoperatively with the Brief Male Sexual Inventory (BSFI). Postoperative data was obtained from those with at least 6 months follow-up data. BSFI scores were also compared to normative controls (derived from the Olmstead County Study of Urinary Symptoms and Health Status among Men). The authors showed increases in all BSFI domains (i.e., sex drive, erection, ejaculation, problem assessment, sexual satisfaction) after surgery. On multivariate analysis, weight loss predicted the degree of improvement in all BSFI domains. The baseline sexual function was lower in the cohort compared to the normative controls in each age group and domain. Postoperative sexual function either approached or equaled those in the normative controls. The authors estimated that "a man who is morbidly obese has the same degree of sexual dysfunction as a nonobese [sic] man about 20 years older" [30].

Diet Studies

A group of investigators from Naples, Italy studied the effect of the Mediterranean diet on erectile function. This diet emphasizes intake of fruits, vegetables, nuts, whole grains, and olive oil. In Esposito et al. [31], 65 men with metabolic syndrome and ED (defined in the study as IIEF-5 ≤ 21) were enrolled in a prospective cohort study for 2 years. The 35 men assigned to the intervention diet were advised to consume at least 250–300 g of fruits, 125–150 g of vegetables, and 25–50 g of nuts per day. They were also encouraged to increase the consumption of olive oil and consume 400 g of whole grains daily. Adherence to diet was assessed by completion of food diaries and meetings with the nutritionist. The 30 men in the control group received general information about healthy food choices but did not receive individualized counseling on dietary modification. At 2 years, men on the Mediterranean diet increased mean IIEF-5 from 14.4 to 18.1; men in the control group had no significant change in IIEF-5. Thirteen men in the interventional group and two in the control group reported an IIEF-5 greater than 21 at the end of the study. When compared to the control group, the interventional group also had improved glycemic and lipid profiles, decreased systolic blood pressure, and decreased C-reactive protein. The interventional group, as expected, also consumed more components of the Mediterranean diet at 2 years compared to baseline.

A similar group of investigators studied the effect of the Mediterranean diet on men with Type 2 diabetes mellitus. In a study by Giugliano et al. [32], 555 men with Type 2 diabetes mellitus completed a food-frequency questionnaire and the IIEF-5. Higher scores on the food-frequency questionnaires denoted higher adherence to the Mediterranean-style diet. Compared to those scoring low on the food-frequency questionnaire, the patients with the highest scores on the food-frequency questionnaire were noted to have lower BMI, waist circumference, waist-to-hip ratio, and lower prevalence of obesity and metabolic syndrome. They also had higher level of physical activity and better glycemic and lipid profiles. The proportion of sexually active men was significantly higher across tertiles of adherence to the Mediterranean diet. Those with the highest scores also were more likely to have significantly lower prevalence of global ED (51.9 % versus 62 %) and severe ED (16.5 % versus 26.4 %).

The relationship between diet and ED was also reported in cross-sectional studies. A survey of 1466 diabetic Canadian men (2011 Survey on Living with Chronic Disease in Canada—Diabetes Component) included questions on ED and the daily consumption of fruits and vegetables [33]. In this group of men, 26.2 % reported having ED (defined as diagnosed by health professional), with the rates increasing with age and duration of diabetes. The rate of ED decreased by 10 % with each increase of 1 serving of fruit or vegetable per day. As a reflection of competing comorbidities, the men with ED also reported "significantly higher rates of hypertension, circulation problems, cardiovascular disease, kidney disease, and nerve damage" [33].

A cross-sectional study of 312 consecutive diabetic men attending a free diabetes clinic in Hamadan, Iran collected demographics, lifestyle factors, comorbidities, medications, diabetes complications, and metabolic control [34]. ED was assessed by IIEF-5. The prevalence of ED was high (94.6%), with 34% representing moderate-to-severe ED. A diet rich in fruits was associated with a lower risk of ED, with an odds ratio of 0.31 for those who consumed fruits daily compared to those who consumed fruits weekly or seldom consumed fruits.

Intensive Lifestyle Changes Studies

To study the effectiveness of weight loss and increased physical activity, 110 obese, sedentary men with ED were enrolled in a RCT for 2 years in Naples, Italy [35]. The study excluded men with diabetes, hypertension, prostatic disease, chronic kidney disease, psychiatric diseases, and/or alcohol/drug abuse. The intervention group ($n = 55$) received advice to reduce caloric intake, dietary counseling with nutritionist, and guidance on physical activity with an exercise trainer. The control group ($n = 55$) were given general information on diet and exercise. After 2 years, mean IIEF-5 improved significantly for the intervention group from 13.9 to 17. There was no change in IIEF-5 for the control group. Of those with improvement in IIEF-5, 17 men in the intervention group and three men in the control group had IIEF-5 greater than 21 after 2 years. On multivariate analysis, BMI, physical activity, and C-reactive protein were independent predictors of IIEF-5 score.

The Look AHEAD (Action for Health in Diabetes) trial was a multicenter RCT that enrolled patients with Type 2 diabetes mellitus, ages 45–74 years, and with an overweight BMI [36]. The sexual ancillary study of this trial recruited 372 male patients from five of the 16 Look AHEAD sites and examined 1-year changes in erectile function. For the ancillary study, the men were either sexually active within the past 6 months of enrollment or were in a committed relationship. The intervention group focused on caloric restriction (e.g., 1200–1500 kcal/day if weight <250 lbs), moderate intensity activity (e.g., brisk walking; 175 min/week), and meetings. The control group received an initial diabetes education course and was invited to three sessions (during year 1) that provided basic education on diet and physical activities. The proportion of ED (defined as IIEF-5 less than 22) at baseline was similar between the two groups (61% of intervention group, 51% of control group). At 1 year, 306 men completed the sexual ancillary study. Those in the intervention group lost significantly more weight (9.9% versus 0.6%) and showed significantly higher fitness level (22.7% versus 4.6%). Eight and 20% of the interventional and control groups reported worsening ED at 1 year. IIEF-5 did improve more for the interventional group (from 17.3 to 18.6) compared to the control group (from 18.3 to 18.4), albeit statistical significance was not present when the data were adjusted for baseline differences ($p = 0.06$). Regression analyses showed that the strongest predictor of the change in erection function was baseline IIEF-5. The percent of weight change was also significantly associated with changes in IIEF-5. In subgroup analysis, those who gained weight reported significant worsening of IIEF-5 over time. There was no dose–response effect present between weight loss and improvement in IIEF-5.

Tobacco Studies

The use of tobacco products has been shown to have an adverse effect on erectile function. In a meta-analysis conducted by Cao et al. [37], which included 4 prospective cohort studies and four case–control studies, the authors summarized the overall odd ratio of ED in prospective cohort studies as 1.51 for current smokers and 1.29 for former smokers. In the Health Professionals Follow-up Study, Bacon et al. [38] assessed for the impact of obesity, physical activity, alcohol use, and smoking on the development of ED. Their analysis considered a subset of men ($n = 22,086$) without major comorbidities and with intact erectile function (described as either *good* or *very good* on the survey) at the beginning of the study in 1986. The last set of questionnaires was given in 2000. In that 14-year time span, 17.7 % of the men reported ED. Smoking and obesity were significantly associated with an increased risk of ED, while physical activity was associated with a decreased risk of ED. For those who developed prostate cancer during follow-up, smoking was also significantly associated with ED.

A prospective study from Iran recruited smokers with ED who had requested nicotine replacement therapy [39]. The investigators excluded those with major comorbidities. Nicotine replacement therapy was given for 1–2 months. Patients (118 ex-smokers, 163 current smokers) were then followed for 1 year. After 1 year, 25 % of the ex-smokers had improvement in the IIEF-5 grade of ED; current smokers showed no improvement. Deterioration in ED grade was seen in 2.5 and 7 % of ex-smokers and current smokers, respectively.

Alcohol Studies

A Western Australian population-based cross-sectional study assessed the association between alcohol consumption and ED [40]. The investigators gathered information on sociodemographic details, erectile function (via IIEF-5), and cardiovascular disease risk factors. The questionnaire also queried the participant's alcohol and tobacco use. Of the 1544 men who answered questions on alcohol use, 87 % were current drinkers, and 6.3 % were former drinkers. Compared to never drinkers, ex-drinkers had higher odds of ED (2.04 when adjusted for age and square of age; 1.22 when additionally adjusted for cardiovascular disease and cigarette smoking). Although not statistically significant, current drinkers had a trend for lower age-adjusted odds of ED compared to never drinkers. When adjusted for cardiovascular disease or cigarette use, the age-adjusted odds of ED for all categories of alcohol drinkers were reduced by 25–30 %.

A meta-analysis by Cheng et al. [41] investigated the risk of ED with different levels of alcohol consumption. This study identified 11 cross-sectional studies that provided adjusted odds ratio for alcohol and analyzed them with a random effects model. None of the studies included men from North America. Regular alcohol consumption was significantly and negatively associated with ED, with an odds ratio of 0.79. Consumption of 8 or more drinks/week was significantly associated with lower risk of ED (odds ratio of 0.85). While the odds ratios were also low, the consumption of less alcohol (i.e., 1–7 drinks/week) was not statistically significant.

Statin Therapy

Gupta et al. [42] performed a systematic review and meta-analysis of RCTs that evaluated the effect of lifestyle interventions and pharmacotherapy for cardiovascular risk factors on the severity of ED. They identified six RCTs, four of which intervene with lifestyle changes that were discussed earlier [21, 31, 35, 36], and two of which intervene with atorvastatin [43, 44]. Meta-analysis of the six RCTs showed a significant improvement in IIEF-5 with a weighted mean difference of 2.66. When pooling the lifestyle intervention and the statin trials separately, they also showed significant improvement in IIEF-5 with weighted mean differences of 2.4 and 3.07, respectively.

Compared to the lifestyle intervention RCTs, the atorvastatin RCTs differ in that they recruited men with ED whose erections responded poorly to sildenafil. In Hermann et al. [43], 12 men with moderate-to-severe ED (defined as IIEF-5 ≤ 16) were randomized to atorvastatin 80 mg ($n=8$) versus placebo ($n=4$) for 12 weeks. Patient recruitment was stopped prematurely because of difficulty with accruing patients and the subsequent availability of additional PDE-5i during the study period. Patients were also prescribed sildenafil 100 mg on-demand during the study. After 12 weeks, mean IIEF-5 increased significantly from 10.3 to 18 for the atorvastatin group. In the placebo patients, the increase in IIEF-5 (from 4 to 12.3) was not statistically significant, with the increase primarily driven by 1 patient with an improvement from 9 to 29.

In Dadkhah et al. [44], 131 men with ED (defined as IIEF-5 ≤ 21) were randomized to atorvastatin 40 mg ($n=66$) versus placebo ($n=65$) for 12 weeks. Patients were also given instructions to take sildenafil 100 mg on-demand during the study. After 12 weeks, the atorvastatin group had a significant increase in IIEF-5 from 10.3 to 13.9. The placebo group showed no overall difference in IIEF-5 after the study. The authors reported a significantly higher proportion of IIEF-5 improvement in the atorvastatin group (37.3 %) compared to placebo group (11.9 %). Four in the atorvastatin group discontinued the medication because of adverse events. The adverse events reported included constipation, dyspepsia, abdominal pain, headache, and myalgia.

A more recent RCT (Erectile Dysfunction and Statins Trial) evaluated the effectiveness of simvastatin in men ≥40 years with untreated ED [45]. The trial randomized 173 men to simvastatin 40 mg ($n=90$) versus placebo ($n=83$). After 6 months, the improvement in IIEF-5 did trend in favor of simvastatin but is not statistically significant (simvastatin vs. placebo: 1.28 vs. 0.07; $p=0.27$). There was a significantly larger improvement in the male ED quality of life score for those on simvastatin compared to placebo. As expected, men on simvastatin had significant reduction on both the 10-year cardiovascular disease risk and low-density lipoprotein level compared to placebo. Of the 126 adverse events reported during the study, none of the 5 serious events were considered related to simvastatin.

Discussion/Conclusions

ED is common worldwide among men and found in higher prevalence with increased age. Patients presenting with ED without a prior diagnosis of cardiovascular disease should undergo cardiovascular evaluation [46]. Many trials have shown that life-style modification, whether it be physical exercise, weight loss, dietary modification, smoking cessation, or a combination thereof, can improve the degree of ED, especially in men with obesity, diabetes, hypertension, and other cardiovascular-related comorbidities [47]. The data on tobacco use and ED support smoking cessation. While there have been no RCTs on alcohol with respect to ED, the meta-analysis does suggest moderate alcohol intake may reduce the risk of ED [41]. The RCTs on statin therapy suggest possible short-term benefit to improving the degree of ED for men who have already tried maximum dose of sildenafil.

To date, there has been no published evidence that supports or refutes the idea of optimizing erectile function in prostate cancer patients prior to radical prostatectomy. Many of the prospective comparison studies on ED risk modification have specifically excluded prostate cancer in their patient selection criteria. Men with ED who can perform these interventions before and after surgery should at least benefit from the interventions' associated cardioprotective effects. Those who are medically unable to perform the interventions are likely already poor/marginal surgical candidates and should consider other options for management of prostate cancer.

Patients on active surveillance for prostate cancer should also consider performing these interventions to improve erectile function. As approximately one-third of those patients do come off protocol [48] and proceed with treatment, they may have sufficient time to implement these interventions (including bariatric surgery, if indicated) to optimize both their erectile function and cardiovascular health.

Overall, the trials on lifestyle modification, tobacco cessation, alcohol use, and statin therapy do not show harmful effect on men with ED and may improve erectile function. Compared to the existing treatment options for ED, these interventions should be able to be implemented at a relatively low cost to patients and should be offered to men with ED, including those with prostate cancer who may later undergo radical prostatectomy for definitive treatment.

References

1. Hatzimouratidis K, Eardley I, Giuliano F, Hatzichristou D, Moncada I, Salonia A, et al. Guidelines on male sexual dysfunction: erectile dysfunction and premature ejaculation. Arnhem: European Association of Urology; 2015. http://uroweb.org/guideline/male-sexual-dysfunction/.

2. Johannes CB, Araujo AB, Feldman HA, Derby CA, Kleinman KP, McKinlay JB. Incidence of erectile dysfunction in men 40 to 69 years old: longitudinal results from the Massachusetts male aging study. J Urol. 2000;163(2):460–3.

3. Laumann EO, Paik A, Rosen RC. Sexual dysfunction in the United States: prevalence and predictors. JAMA. 1999;281(6):537–44.

4. Lewis RW, Fugl-Meyer KS, Corona G, Hayes RD, Laumann EO, Moreira Jr ED, et al. Definitions/epidemiology/risk factors for sexual dysfunction. J Sex Med. 2010;7(4 Pt 2): 1598–607.

5. Rosen RC, Riley A, Wagner G, Osterloh IH, Kirkpatrick J, Mishra A. The international index of erectile function (IIEF): a multidimensional scale for assessment of erectile dysfunction. Urology. 1997;49(6):822–30.

6. Rosen RC, Cappelleri JC, Smith MD, Lipsky J, Pena BM. Development and evaluation of an abridged, 5-item version of the International Index of Erectile Function (IIEF-5) as a diagnostic tool for erectile dysfunction. Int J Impot Res. 1999;11(6):319–26.

7. Cappelleri JC, Rosen RC. The Sexual Health Inventory for Men (SHIM): a 5-year review of research and clinical experience. Int J Impot Res. 2005;17(4):307–19.

8. O'Leary MP, Fowler FJ, Lenderking WR, Barber B, Sagnier PP, Guess HA, et al. A brief male sexual function inventory for urology. Urology. 1995;46(5):697–706.

9. Glick HA, McCarron TJ, Althof SE, Corty EW, Willke RJ. Construction of scales for the Center for Marital and Sexual Health (CMASH) Sexual Functioning Questionnaire. J Sex Marital Ther. 1997;23(2):103–17.

10. Clayton AH, McGarvey EL, Clavet GJ. The Changes in Sexual Functioning Questionnaire (CSFQ): development, reliability, and validity. Psychopharmacol Bull. 1997;33(4):731–45.

11. Althof SE, Corty EW, Levine SB, Levine F, Burnett AL, McVary K, et al. EDITS: development of questionnaires for evaluating satisfaction with treatments for erectile dysfunction. Urology. 1999;53(4):793–9.

12. Rosen RC, Catania J, Pollack L, Althof S, O'Leary M, Seftel AD. Male Sexual Health Questionnaire (MSHQ): scale development and psychometric validation. Urology. 2004;64(4):777–82.

13. Mulhall JP, King R, Kirby M, Hvidsten K, Symonds T, Bushmakin AG, et al. Evaluating the sexual experience in men: validation of the sexual experience questionnaire. J Sex Med. 2008;5(2):365–76.

14. Shamloul R, Ghanem H. Erectile dysfunction. Lancet. 2013;381(9861):153–65.

15. Masters WH, Johnson VE. Human sexual response. Boston, MA: Little, Brown & Company; 1965.

16. Lizza EF, Rosen RC. Definition and classification of erectile dysfunction: report of the Nomenclature Committee of the International Society of Impotence Research. Int J Impot Res. 1999;11(3):141–3.

17. Selvin E, Burnett AL, Platz EA. Prevalence and risk factors for erectile dysfunction in the US. Am J Med. 2007;120(2):151–7.

18. Francis ME, Kusek JW, Nyberg LM, Eggers PW. The contribution of common medical conditions and drug exposures to erectile dysfunction in adult males. J Urol. 2007;178(2):591–6. discussion 596.

19. Dong JY, Zhang YH, Qin LQ. Erectile dysfunction and risk of cardiovascular disease: meta-analysis of prospective cohort studies. J Am Coll Cardiol. 2011;58(13):1378–85.

20. Cheng JY, Ng EM, Ko JS, Chen RY. Physical activity and erectile dysfunction: meta-analysis of population-based studies. Int J Impot Res. 2007;19(3):245–52.

21. Lamina S, Okoye CG, Dagogo TT. Therapeutic effect of an interval exercise training program in the management of erectile dysfunction in hypertensive patients. J Clin Hypertens (Greenwich). 2009;11(3):125–9.

22. La Vignera S, Condorelli R, Vicari E, D'Agata R, Calogero A. Aerobic physical activity improves endothelial function in the middle-aged patients with erectile dysfunction. Aging Male. 2011;14(4):265–72.

23. Maio G, Saraeb S, Marchiori A. Physical activity and PDE5 inhibitors in the treatment of erectile dysfunction: results of a randomized controlled study. J Sex Med. 2010;7(6):2201–8.

24. Bacon CG, Mittleman MA, Kawachi I, Giovannucci E, Glasser DB, Rimm EB. Sexual function in men older than 50 years of age: results from the health professionals follow-up study. Ann Intern Med. 2003;139(3):161–8.
25. Kratzik CW, Schatzl G, Lunglmayr G, Rucklinger E, Huber J. The impact of age, body mass index and testosterone on erectile dysfunction. J Urol. 2005;174(1):240–3.
26. Khoo J, Piantadosi C, Worthley S, Wittert GA. Effects of a low-energy diet on sexual function and lower urinary tract symptoms in obese men. Int J Obes (Lond). 2010;34(9):1396–403.
27. Khoo J, Piantadosi C, Duncan R, Worthley SG, Jenkins A, Noakes M, et al. Comparing effects of a low-energy diet and a high-protein low-fat diet on sexual and endothelial function, urinary tract symptoms, and inflammation in obese diabetic men. J Sex Med. 2011;8(10):2868–75.
28. Khoo J, Ling PS, Tan J, Teo A, Ng HL, Chen RY, et al. Comparing the effects of meal replacements with reduced-fat diet on weight, sexual and endothelial function, testosterone and quality of life in obese Asian men. Int J Impot Res. 2014;26(2):61–6.
29. Reis LO, Favaro WJ, Barreiro GC, de Oliveira LC, Chaim EA, Fregonesi A, et al. Erectile dysfunction and hormonal imbalance in morbidly obese male is reversed after gastric bypass surgery: a prospective randomized controlled trial. Int J Androl. 2010;33(5):736–44.
30. Dallal RM, Chernoff A, O'Leary MP, Smith JA, Braverman JD, Quebbemann BB. Sexual dysfunction is common in the morbidly obese male and improves after gastric bypass surgery. J Am Coll Surg. 2008;207(6):859–64.
31. Esposito K, Ciotola M, Giugliano F, De Sio M, Giugliano G, D'armiento M, et al. Mediterranean diet improves erectile function in subjects with the metabolic syndrome. Int J Impot Res. 2006;18(4):405–10.
32. Giugliano F, Maiorino MI, Bellastella G, Autorino R, De Sio M, Giugliano D, et al. Adherence to Mediterranean diet and erectile dysfunction in men with type 2 diabetes. J Sex Med. 2010;7(5).1911–7.
33. Wang F, Dai S, Wang M, Morrison H. Erectile dysfunction and fruit/vegetable consumption among diabetic Canadian men. Urology. 2013;82(6):1330–5.
34. Shiri R, Ansari M, Falah Hassani K. Association between comorbidity and erectile dysfunction in patients with diabetes. Int J Impot Res. 2006;18(4):348–53.
35. Esposito K, Giugliano F, Di Palo C, Giugliano G, Marfella R, D'Andrea F, et al. Effect of lifestyle changes on erectile dysfunction in obese men: a randomized controlled trial. JAMA. 2004;291(24):2978–84.
36. Wing RR, Rosen RC, Fava JL, Bahnson J, Brancati F, Gendrano Iii IN, et al. Effects of weight loss intervention on erectile function in older men with type 2 diabetes in the Look AHEAD trial. J Sex Med. 2010;7(1 Pt 1):156–65.
37. Cao S, Yin X, Wang Y, Zhou H, Song F, Lu Z. Smoking and risk of erectile dysfunction: systematic review of observational studies with meta-analysis. PLoS One. 2013;8(4), e60443.
38. Bacon CG, Mittleman MA, Kawachi I, Giovannucci E, Glasser DB, Rimm EB. A prospective study of risk factors for erectile dysfunction. J Urol. 2006;176(1):217–21.
39. Pourmand G, Alidaee MR, Rasuli S, Maleki A, Mehrsai A. Do cigarette smokers with erectile dysfunction benefit from stopping? A prospective study. BJU Int. 2004;94(9):1310–3.
40. Chew KK, Bremner A, Stuckey B, Earle C, Jamrozik K. Alcohol consumption and male erectile dysfunction: an unfounded reputation for risk? J Sex Med. 2009;6(5):1386–94.
41. Cheng JY, Ng EM, Chen RY, Ko JS. Alcohol consumption and erectile dysfunction: meta-analysis of population-based studies. Int J Impot Res. 2007;19(4):343–52.
42. Gupta BP, Murad MH, Clifton MM, Prokop L, Nehra A, Kopecky SL. The effect of lifestyle modification and cardiovascular risk factor reduction on erectile dysfunction: a systematic review and meta-analysis. Arch Intern Med. 2011;171(20):1797–803.
43. Herrmann HC, Levine LA, Macaluso Jr J, Walsh M, Bradbury D, Schwartz S, et al. Can atorvastatin improve the response to sildenafil in men with erectile dysfunction not initially responsive to sildenafil? Hypothesis and pilot trial results. J Sex Med. 2006;3(2):303–8.
44. Dadkhah F, Safarinejad MR, Asgari MA, Hosseini SY, Lashay A, Amini E. Atorvastatin improves the response to sildenafil in hypercholesterolemic men with erectile dysfunction not initially responsive to sildenafil. Int J Impot Res. 2010;22(1):51–60.

45. Trivedi D, Kirby M, Wellsted DM, Ali S, Hackett G, O'Connor B, et al. Can simvastatin improve erectile function and health-related quality of life in men aged >/=40 years with erectile dysfunction? Results of the Erectile Dysfunction and Statins Trial [ISRCTN66772971. BJU Int. 2013;111(2):324–33.
46. Kostis JB, Jackson G, Rosen R, Barrett-Connor E, Billups K, Burnett AL, et al. Sexual dysfunction and cardiac risk (the Second Princeton Consensus Conference). Am J Cardiol. 2005;96(2):313–21.
47. Maiorino MI, Bellastella G, Esposito K. Lifestyle modifications and erectile dysfunction: what can be expected? Asian J Androl. 2015;17(1):5–10.
48. Klotz L. Active surveillance for low-risk prostate cancer. Curr Urol Rep. 2015; 16(4):24-015-0492-z.

Chapter 4
Pathophysiology of Nerve Injury and Its Effect on Return of Erectile Function

Louis Eichel, Douglas Skarecky, and Thomas E. Ahlering

Introduction

Dr. Patrick Walsh and his associates initiated the concept of attempting to preserve sexual potency following a radical prostatectomy (RP) when they originally described the anatomy of the cavernous nerves (CN) and the process of anatomical nerve-sparing radical prostatectomy [1, 2]. However, two decades passed until new surgical technology introduced the possibility of a near bloodless surgical field and dramatically improved visualization via laparoscopic and robotic radical prostatectomy popularized by Vallencien, Guilloneau, Abbou, and indeed many of the authors of this book. With these less invasive surgical approaches surgeons were better able to apply the principles of visual nerve preservation with retrograde and antegrade nerve-sparing approaches. However, anatomical preservation although critically important has and does not explain how or why potency recovery takes 2 years. The foundation of our modern understanding of nerve injury and healing originated with Sir Herbert Seddon in the 1940s who demonstrated the pathophysiology of injury and recovery in peripheral nerves [3]. Seddon's discoveries became the basis for many subsequent discoveries in the field of neuropathology and have also proven to be the basis upon which modern techniques of nerve preservation and reconstruction are based for various surgeries. Indeed, the application of Seddon's principles to the injury and recovery of function of the CN was only introduced in 2008. Clearly, basic neurosurgical concepts such as "dissecting the organ off of the nerve

L. Eichel, M.D.
Division of Urology, Rochester General Hospital, Rochester, NY, USA

Center for Urology, 2615 Culver Rd, Ste 100, Rochester, NY 14609, USA

D. Skarecky, B.S. • T.E. Ahlering, MD (✉)
Department of Urology, Irvine Medical Center, University of California, Irvine, 333 The City Drive West, Suite 2100, RT 81, Orange, CA 92868, USA
e-mail: tahlerin@uci.edu

© Springer International Publishing Switzerland 2016
S. Razdan (ed.), *Urinary Continence and Sexual Function After Robotic Radical Prostatectomy*, DOI 10.1007/978-3-319-39448-0_4

as opposed to dissecting the nerve off of the organ" originated from these seminal works. In as much as this has been a challenge, the major advances of magnified, 3D, high definition vision systems integrated with highly dexterous, robotic, micro-surgical instrumentation have also provided many opportunities to advance our understanding of reducing "injury" to the CN while visualizing and preserving it. This chapter summarizes the basic anatomy and more importantly the pathophysiol-ogy of cavernous nerve injury and how our expanding knowledge of this topic will lead to future improvement of clinical outcomes.

Potency Outcomes Self-Assessment

The most critical component required for assessment and subsequent understanding of sexual outcomes following RP is obsessive collection and collation of validated self-reported baseline and follow-up questionnaires. The primary reason surgeons do not improve outcomes is the lack of personal experience and the uninformed assumption of "acceptable" results. It is imperative for the robotic surgeon to estab-lish a surgical database of preoperative demographics and postoperative outcomes for critical self-evaluation. Self-assessment is a continual iterative process, and as the volume of ones cases increases, a personal database allows one to measure outcomes against published results. Through the process of self-assessment of out-comes, the surgeon can determine if there are specific troublesome technical or clinical issues. There are two important self-assessment tools: rigorous data collec-tion and reviewing personal and "expert" video recordings.

The collection of data regarding patients' baseline demographics, intra and post-operative outcomes is essential. Preoperative data must be stringently collected as most functional outcomes are dependent on the baseline characteristics. A proposed minimum data collection design is a baseline International Index of Erectile Function (IIEF-5) also known as SHIM (Sex Health Index in Men), age, medical issues such as hypertension and diabetes, and testosterone levels (free and total). At baseline, Rosen et al. [4] demonstrated that an IIEF-5 score of 22–25 was highly predictive of normal erectile function. In our experience we have not seen a single case of recovery of sexual function following radical prostatectomy if the baseline IIEF-5 is below 15. Additionally, if a patient is dependent on a PDE inhibitor to achieve a given IIEF-5 score we recommend subtracting seven points to establish baseline function. Postoperative oncologic and continence data, in addition to com-plication rates, should be meticulously recorded to improve surgical technique and identify areas that may lead to improvements in patient outcomes.

Defining "recovery" of potency continues to be practically and theoretically a real challenge. Some authors arbitrarily define or recommend an IIEF-5 score of >16, 21, or 25 with or without PDEi; some attempt to simplify the matter by defining recovered potency as a patient reporting a score of 3 or higher for question 5 of the IIEF-5[4–7]. We suggest a quantitative and a qualitative assessment (Fig. 4.1). We define potency quantitatively (with or without PDE5 inhibitors) as an affirmative answer to 2 questions from EPIC questionnaire, (1) "Are your erections adequate

1. Do you presently have erections firm enough for penetration **Yes / No**   Are they Satisfactory? **Yes / No**
2. Please circle the fullness you are able to achieve in your erections compared to before surgery?
3. **0%**   **10 %**   **25%**   **50%**   **75%**   **85%**   **90%**   **95%**   **100%**
4. Do you currently use any medications listed for potency? If Very Helpful-**VH**, if Slightly Helpful-**SH**, if Not Helpful-**NH**
   Viagra_____ Levitra_____ Cialis_____ Muse_____ Other_____
   _____ None
5. If you have taken Viagra or Cialis, please describe: Daily Yes/No   As Needed   Yes/No

Date started _____ and **for how many weeks**_____

1. How do you rate your confidence that you could get and keep an erection?

Very low	Low	Moderate	High	Very High
1	2	3	4	5

2. When you had erections with sexual stimulation, how often were your erections hard enough for penetration (entering your partner).

No sexual activity	Almost never or never	A few times (less than half the time)	Sometimes (about half the time)	Most times (much more than half the time)	Almost Always Or Always
0	1	2	3	4	5

3. During sexual intercourse, how often were you able to maintain your erection after you had penetrated (entered) your partner?

Did not Attempt intercourse	Almost never or never	A few times (less than half the time)	Sometimes (about half the time)	Most times (much more than half the time)	Almost Always Or Always
0	1	2	3	4	5

4. During sexual intercourse, how difficult was it to maintain your erection to completion of intercourse?

Did not attempt intercourse	Extremely Difficult	Very Difficult	Difficult	Slightly Difficult	Not Difficult
0	1	2	3	4	5

5. When you attempted sexual intercourse, how often was it satisfactory to you?

Did not attempt intercourse	Almost never or never	A few times (less than half the time)	Sometimes (about half the time)	Most times (much more than half the time)	Almost Always Or Always
0	1	2	3	4	5

SCORE_____

Fig. 4.1 IIEF-5 and quantitative and qualitative sexual function assessment used for pre and post-operative assessment of potency

for vaginal penetration?" and (2) "Are your erections satisfactory?"[8]. For qualitative assessment we recommend the IIEF-5. Additionally, we have found that simply asking the patient what percent of their baseline erectile function they have regained postoperatively can be most helpful, especially in the early months following surgery when erections are not adequate (Fig. 4.1 question 3).

Recording case videos can be extremely advantageous to not only the novice surgeon but those with experience as well. Reviewing ones procedure is particularly useful for difficult cases and for cases with excellent functional outcomes.

Gross Anatomic Studies of the Cavernous Nerves

The anatomic basis for erectile function [1] and the subsequent technique for nerve-sparing radical retropubic prostatectomy were initially described by Walsh and associates in 1983 [2]. The authors described the pathways of the parasympathetic

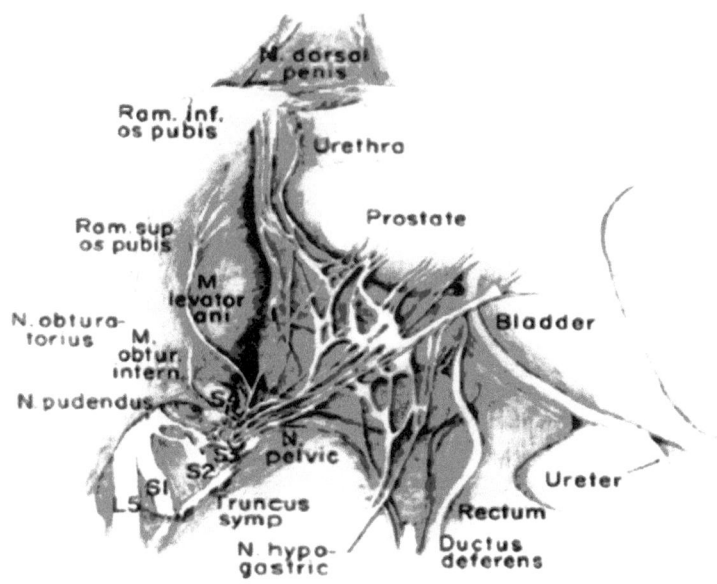

Fig. 4.2 Anatomic drawing depicting the path of the cavernous nerves taken with permission from the authors. Walsh, P.C. and Donker, P.J., Impotence following radical prostatectomy: insight into etiology and prevention. J Urol, 1982. 128(3): p. 492–7

nerves that emanate from the spinal cord, S2–S4, through the hypogastric plexus past the tips of the seminal vesicles along side the rectum and then along the posterolateral aspect of the prostate between the true capsule and the lateral prostatic fascia finally piercing the urogenital diaphragm just posterior and lateral to the urethra (Fig. 4.2). Widespread popularization of this knowledge has facilitated our ability to preserve the cavernous nerves. Since this landmark study other studies have led to the discovery of additional findings potentially related to the physical preservation of the nerves.

Takenaka and associates have contributed several papers regarding male pelvic neuroanatomy. In two studies, they performed gross and histologic dissections of male cadavers defining the cranial and caudal paths of the cavernous nerves [9, 10]. With regard to the origin of the nerves, they determined that in most individuals the traditional neurovascular bundles contain few parasympathetic nerve components proximal to the bladder–prostate junction. Instead, parasympathetic nerve branches configured in a "spray-like" distribution approach the dorsolateral prostate at least 20 mm below the bladder–prostate junction.

In another paper, Takenaka and associates describe the presence of autonomic ganglion cells which were postulated to have an effect on the return of potency [11]. Ganglion cells were found throughout the surfaces of the pelvic viscera including the hypogastric plexus, the seminal vesicles, the levator ani muscle, the bladder, and the prostate. The NVB also contained many ganglion cells. The number and distribution varied a great deal and the authors' speculated this variability might contribute to susceptibility or resistance to impotence. However, it has historically been recognized that these ganglia correspond to the end organs they are adjacent to and don't have any bearing on potency whatsoever [12]. In fact, Alsaid et al. described the presence of various types of nerve fibers within the NVBs in the male fetus. Using 3D modeling, they found that multiple types of nerve fibers originated from the inferior hypogastric plexus, providing cholinergic, adrenergic, and sensory innervation to seminal vesicles, vas deferens, prostate, and urethral sphincter in a fan-like formation [13]. Interestingly, similar studies by Menon and Tewari have shown that the pelvic plexus is located [14, 15] midway adjacent to the tip of the seminal vesicle. These authors like Takenaka also described the appearance of multiple autonomic ganglia in the vicinity of the cavernous nerves. Both describe interconnections between the left and right neurovascular bundles along the anterior rectal wall within Denonvillier's fascia. Unlike Takenaka, however Tewari and associates describe cavernous branches of the pelvic plexus coalescing to form a more traditional "bundle" that runs within a triangular area (the neurovascular triangle) between the inner and outer layers of the periprostatic fascia and Denonvillier's fascia. The inner layer of periprostatic fascia (also called as the prostatic fascia) forms the medial vertical wall of this triangle; the outer layer of periprostatic fascia (also called as lateral pelvic fascia) forms the lateral wall, and the posterior wall of this triangle is formed by the anterior layer of Denonvillier's fascia. This triangular space is wide near the base of the prostate and becomes narrower near the apex. Menon has described a belief that additional nerves important for sexual function exist within periprostatic fascia that covers the lateral and anterior surface of the prostate that he aptly named the Veil of Aphrodite. The authors acknowledge they have not traced these nerves to the corpora cavernosa. They also hypothesize that because the plane of dissection is away from the cavernosal nerves other factors such as decreased traction, avoidance of thermal injury, and preservation of extra blood supply may play a role in preservation of nerve function.

In 2005, Costello and associates reported a detailed description of the plexus of nerves running within the NVB [16]. They found multiple nerve branches that emanated from the hypogastric plexus and spread significantly, with up to 3 cm separating the anterior and posterior nerves (Fig. 4.3). Similar to Menon, Costello noted that the NVB courses along the posterolateral border of the prostate within the bounds of lateral pelvic fascia, the pararectal fascia, and Denonvillier's fascia. In distinction to Menon and associates, they felt that the nerves located within the Veil of Aphrodite primarily innervate the prostate. This finding was more recently confirmed by Ganzer et al. who used immunohistochemical staining to ascertain the type and distribution of the periprostatic nerves. They found that parasympathetic (pro erectile) nerves were most prevalent dorsolaterally (within the true neurovascular bundle) with minimal percentages of fibers more anterolaterally on the prostate [17]. Similar to Takenaka, Costello found that the nerves converge mid prostate forming a more condensed bundle and then diverge again when approaching the prostatic apex where they divide into numerous small branches that descend along the posterolateral aspect of the membranous urethra, before penetrating the corpora cavernosa.

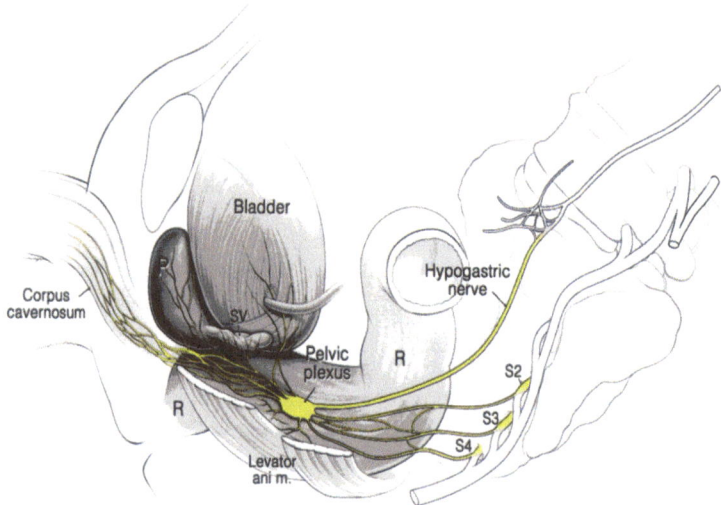

Fig. 4.3 Anatomic drawing of the path of the cavernous nerves based on cadaveric dissection. Note the posterolateral position of the neurovascular bundle in relation to the prostate. The nerve fibers more anterior on the prostatic surface do not go to the corpora cavernosum. Taken with permission from the authors. Costello, A.J., M. Brooks, and O.J. Cole, *Anatomical studies of the neurovascular bundle and cavernosal nerves*. BJU Int, 2004. 94(7): p. 1071–6

From the surgeon's perspective there are several take-home messages to be gained from these important anatomic studies: First, the most obvious and helpful landmark to identify the neurovascular bundle is the prostatic vascular pedicle (PVP). Transection of the PVP should be performed with care. This is the first point where surgical trauma caused by thermal injury (excessive cautery), traction (via dissection for clip placement), or direct transection risks collateral injury to the NVB. The authors share several helpful observations regarding the minimization of cautery and traction later in this chapter. Once the PVP is transected the NVB is posterior and lateral to the prostatic surface running along the side of the rectum extending from the base to the apex. It is our opinion that the inadvertent permanent transection of the NVB occurs most frequently at the apex slightly posterior and lateral to the urethra where the structure is most delicate. Dissection of tissues anterior to the urethra (dorsal venous complex and puboprostatic ligaments) does not risk NVB injury.

Pathophysiology of Cavernous Nerve Injury

With the above information regarding the anatomy of the neurovascular bundles in mind it is also important to consider the microscopic anatomy of these nerves and how this relates to nerve injury and healing. The peripheral nervous system is comprised of somatic motor nerves, sensory nerves, and autonomic nerves (parasympathetic or sympathetic). The parasympathetic nerves are responsible for erectile function. Although the name "autonomic" implies that this system functions in an isolated manner, the autonomic system relies on sensory information received from both the peripheral and central nervous system [18]. Erectile function is governed by the parasympathetic nervous system (PNS). All parasympathetic pathways consist of two neurons (the preganglionic neuron and the postganglionic neuron). The cell body of the efferent preganglionic neurons originates in the gray matter of the spinal chord and leave the central nervous system via the spinal nerves. In the case of erectile function, the preganglionic parasympathetic nerves leave the spinal chord via the S2–S4 spinal nerves and then travel to the pelvic plexus. It is generally recorded that parasympathetic preganglionic nerves are long and synapse within a second ganglion on the organ (i.e., corporal bodies) and then the postganglionic fibers travel via short nerves (2–3 mm) to innervate the penis. Currently, there is controversy regarding this matter, however, ultrastructural and functional studies of the cavernous nerves in rats have shown that the cavernous nerves contain both myelinated and nonmyelinated fibers and that most myelinated fibers within the cavernous nerves are preganglionic parasympathetic fibers [19]. Hence, it is reasonable to say that this also most likely the case in humans.

Preganglionic fibers are myelinated and postganglionic fibers are nonmyelinated. The distinction between pre and postganglionic parasympathetic fibers anatomically is that each individual axon of a preganglionic fiber is associated with a single Schwann cell that envelopes it in a myelin sheath whereas for postganglionic fibers multiple axons are enveloped by a single Schwann cell. *It is important to note that both myelinated and nonmyelinated nerves have the ability to heal and regenerate because they are both housed by Schwann cells and can both heal and regenerate* as described later [20, 21].

Definitions of Nerve Injury

During World War II, Sir Herbert Seddon defined peripheral nerve injuries into three categories of brutality [3]. The least severe, designated neurapraxia was considered a mild injury due to nerve contusion from blunt impact or stretch injury to the nerve without structural damage (Fig. 4.4, top). This concussion-like state is caused by damage to the perineural blood supply and results in a short-lived conduction block allowing full recovery in days to weeks.

The second level of injury, axonotmesis is the result of axonal disruption and Wallerian degeneration; however, the perineurium is preserved and the nerve or axon retains the ability to regenerate from the point of injury to the end organ provided the perineurium remains intact (Fig. 4.4, middle). Again, both myelinated and unmyelinated fibers can undergo axonal sprouting and regenerate [20]. Notably, regrowth of the axon advances at ≈1 mm/day or 2.54 cm/month and recovery takes 8–24 months. In this case the role of the microenvironment within which the axons are regenerating is critical and may be a potential source for augmentation by the addition of chemical or physical agents that promote regeneration.

The most severe of the three classifications and the most grim nerve injury to overcome is neurotmesis, a severe injury or a laceration that completely cuts across the axon and

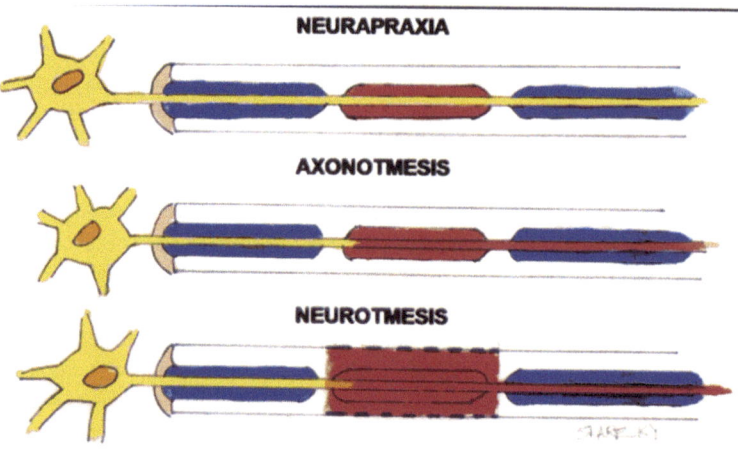

Fig. 4.4 Drawing depicting the three types of nerve injury described by Sir Herbert Seddon

perineurium, providing no scaffolding for regrowth of the axon, and generally resulting in a neuroma or scar (Fig. 4.4, bottom). With this more severe form of injury there is a greater chance of neuronal death and hence little capacity for regrowth of the axon.

Thermal Mechanisms for Cavernous Nerve Injury

The use of thermal energy to control the PVP is now a well-recognized mechanism of NVB damage as the NVB resides millimeters posterior-lateral to the PVP. In the early years of robotic and laparoscopic prostatectomy, the vascular pedicles were most commonly controlled with various types of cautery. Typically bipolar cautery would be used followed by cutting with scissors. This approach of cauterizing and cutting leads to substantial desiccation and thermal spread which in turn caused varying degrees of nerve injury. Early in our experience, we reported the adoption of a thermal technique to control the PVP using temporary occlusion of the PVP with bulldog clamps followed by suture ligation [22]. By simply avoiding cautery, potency at 3 months increased from 8 to 38 % [23, 24]. Remarkably, there was also a slow and steady recovery of potency in the cautery group over 2 years[25]. The best explanation for this delay was that although some injury to the NVB occurred, the injury was not permanent and the cavernosal nerves regenerated and potency was recovered (Fig. 4.5).

The reasons for the 2-year period needed for recovery of erections is rooted in basic and clinical science. Temperature increases of just 4 °C (heating tissue from 37 to 41 °C) can produce neural injury [26, 27]. Reaching temperatures of 45–60 °C causes more damaging protein denaturation and temperatures above this level cause protein coagulation which induces cell death [26]. It has been demonstrated that electrocautery produces temperature elevations and thermal energy effects beyond

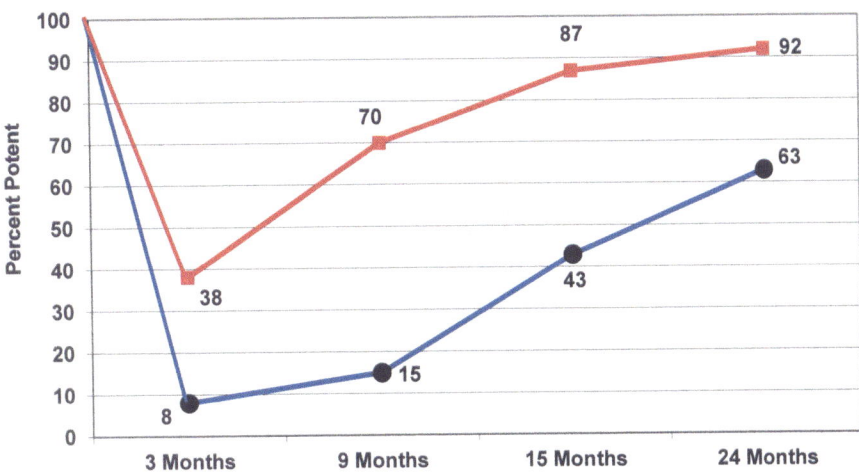

Fig. 4.5 Potency rates for patients in the author's series at 3, 9, 15, and 24 months following robotic radical prostatectomy. The *blue line* represents patients for whom cautery was used to secure the prostatic vascular pedicle with obvious resultant injury, however at 2 years recovery was substantial. The *red line* represents the authors "cautery free" technique to secure the prostatic vascular pedicle

the site of cautery. In essence standard laws of thermodynamics apply. Donzelli and associates demonstrated that both monopolar and bipolar cautery cause thermal injury to nearby neural tissue [28]. The importance of thermal injury to the caverno-sal nerve was demonstrated in a landmark paper by Ong and associates that described the effects of thermal injury in a canine model [29]. In this study, monopolar elec-trocautery, bipolar electrocautery, and harmonic shears all resulted in a >95 % decrease in cavernosal pressures to standard suture ligatures for unilateral caverno-sal nerve dissection. Histologic studies comparing the individual groups confirmed an increased amount of inflammation associated with the use of heat. Mandhani and colleagues measured temperature changes at the NVB with monopolar and bipolar cautery during robotic prostatectomy. The authors found that both mono and bipolar electrocautery raise temperatures to an equivalent degree but that monopolar cau-tery appears to coagulate more efficiently and hence shorter periods of application at lower temperatures are necessary [30]. Another interesting study by Khan and associates demonstrated the thermodynamic impact of heat sink effect by adjacent arteries and veins (Fig. 4.6). These authors demonstrated that thermal energy applied adjacent to inferior epigastric vessels had minimal temperature spread [31]. Zorn and colleagues also nicely demonstrated that the pathological findings of thermal spread to adjacent tissues can be measurably reduced by using cold irrigation concomitantly with cautery [32]. The authors have found that using cold irrigation to limit thermal spread of monopolar cautery has allowed us to reduce the amount of traction needed during PVP transection. Instead of applying clips or suture liga-tures to the PVP, the authors simply recommend suture ligation or if the pedicle is too thick to simply cut the PVP. The highly magnified view presented during robotic

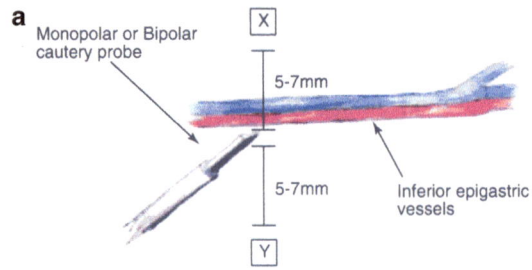

X - Temperature probe with intervening vessels,
    5-7mm from the cautery tip

Y - Temperature probe without intervening
    vessels, 5-7mm from the cautery tip

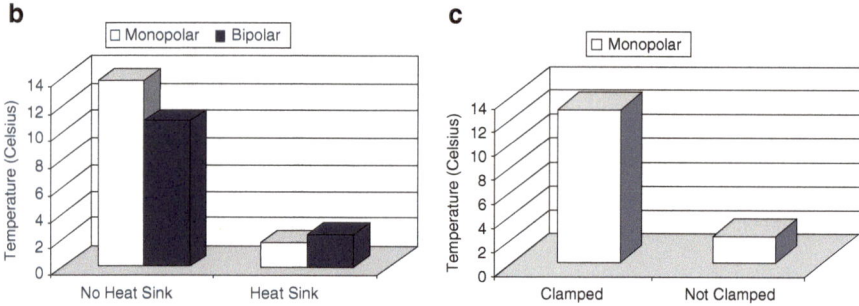

Fig. 4.6 (**a**) Application of monopolar or bipolar cautery at 20 W with (*x* distance) and without (*y* distance) intervening inferior epigastric vessels. (**b**) With interposing inferior epigastric vessels (heat sink), thermal spread is markedly reduced at 5–7 mm from monopolar or bipolar cautery probe. (**c**) With the interposing inferior epigastric vessels clamped, thermal spread across the vessels is markedly increased at 5–7 mm from the MP cautery probe, eliminating the 'heat sink' affect. Figures taken from: Khan, F., et al., *Spread of thermal energy and heat sinks: implications for nerve-sparing robotic prostatectomy*. J Endourol, 2007. 21(10): p. 1195–8

prostatectomy along with copious cold irrigation allows individual bleeders to be identified. The use of very judicious spot monopolar cautery can be used to control these bleeders while minimizing thermal spread to the NVB.

Traction Mechanisms for Cavernous Nerve Injury and the Application of Minimally Invasive Traction (MIT)

From 2003 to 2005 the transition to a thermal technique for transecting the PVP during robotic prostatectomy was reported using temporary occlusion of the PVP with a bulldog clamp [23]. The development of "cautery free" techniques certainly enhanced potency outcomes compared to previous results with cautery. However, even with totally energy free surgery, at least 65 % of men take 9–15 months to recover erectile function [8]. The reason for this phenomenon must be injury due to traction [33]. There are competing goals during radical prostatectomy. The principles of "traction and countertraction" are important in terms of surgical exposure and performing and anatomically correct dissection. On the other hand, these principles are in direct opposition to the neurosurgical premise of "dissecting the tumor off of the nerve." This basic premise of neurosurgery has been known and taught for decades to avoid undue nerve injuries during procedures across all surgical disciplines.

Excessive traction on the neurovascular bundle must have profound unintended consequences as the NVB is quite fragile. Traction injury may occur by direct stretching of the nerves or because of microvascular bleeding in the perineurium leading to secondary infiltration, compression, and inflammation. Figure 4.7 depicts the next technical/surgical hurdle to overcome for preserving potency postradical prostatectomy. It is the mastery of Minimally Invasive Traction (MIT). Similar to other specialties in which "dissecting the tumor off of the nerve" is instilled from day 1, we as robotic surgeons must turn our concentration toward minimizing traction during ligation of the PVP and dissection of the NVB. This remains a particularly challenging dissection for the experienced surgeon and a formidable obstacle for the novice.

Much has been written about avoiding cautery during NVB preservation. Indeed, a 2012 consensus RARP group recommended that the simplest solution is to avoid thermal energy altogether near the NVB [34]. Although complete avoidance of cautery has its stated advantages this method necessitates the use of clips or ligatures which again requires tissue on tension to apply. How then does one avoid tension and minimize damage from cautery. It is possible to minimize traction by simply cutting through the PVP with cold scissors. With regard to control of bleeding when this is done, there is evidence that if the laws of thermodynamics are observed, cautery can be applied while keeping thermal spread to a minimum [31]. This is accomplished by using low wattage, short bursts of cautery performed in a pinpoint fashion and maximizing distance from the NVB. The addition of cooled saline irrigation may further

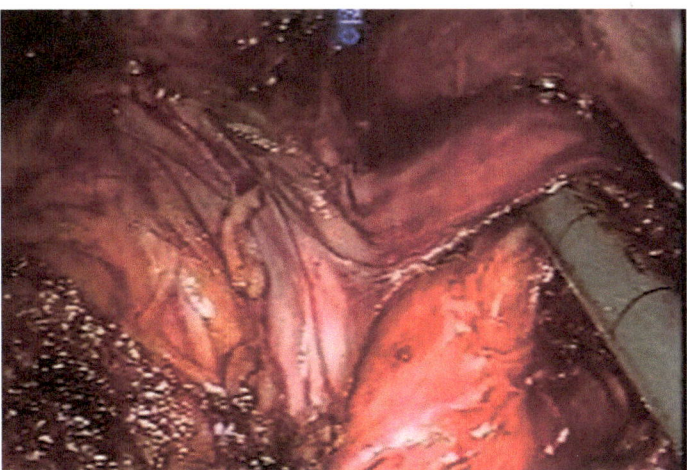

Fig. 4.7 For mastery of Minimally Invasive Traction (MIT), robotic surgeons must turn their concentration toward minimizing traction during ligation of the PVP and dissection of the NVB, by "dissecting the tumor off of the nerve," and avoid the opposite as shown in this figure

limit the spread of heat from surgery [32]. It remains to be seen if such modifications will lead to improved outcomes but certainly we must place emphasis on these basic neurosurgical principles and adapt our technique to minimize nerve injury.

Nerve Redundancy

A very intriguing and important question is what evidence exists regarding the critical volume or percentage of nerve required for preservation of potency? Simply put: What impact does widely excising one of the NVBs have on potency? The fact that there is any recovery speaks to "systems redundancy." We compared potency outcomes in patients in whom we spared both nerves (BNS) to those who had one excised UNS [35]. Also queried was the qualitative recovery following preservation of one versus two nerves, i.e., a doubling of nerve volume. Definitions of unilateral nerve sparing were quite specific; it only included patients with a wide excision of one nerve, which was confirmed pathologically. The group of men undergoing bilateral nerve preservation had a 2-year recovery rate of 92 % whereas men having just one nerve preserved recovered 80 % of the time. So with a 50% reduction of nerve tissue the potency rate was only diminished by approximately 15 %. Qualitatively for the 80% of men reporting successful erections after UNS the average postoperative IIEF-5 scores were not significantly different (UNS 22.0 vs BNS 21.0).

Similar findings have been reported by Walsh and colleagues [36]. They reported that 69 % of men potent before RP who had unilateral wide excision were potent after RP, compared to 85 % who had BNS. Kundu and associates reported a similar trend in overall potency rates at 18 months, of 53 and 76 % after UNS and BNS RP, respectively [37]. What is consistent across all these reports is that doubling the volume of nerve tissue improved potency rates by about 1.15–1.4×. This finding supports redundancy and also speaks against using extreme measures such as intrafascial nerve-sparing dissection. For example, intrafascial dissection might preserve another 5 % of nerve tissue but, considering the data earlier, the benefits to increased potency would only rise minimally if at all.

Testosterone

The negative impact of hypogonadism has been called "The Dark side of Testosterone Deficiency" and manifests as cardiovascular and stroke disease, Type 2 diabetes, metabolic syndrome, central obesity, lack of energy, and erectile dysfunction [38]. Defining hypogonadal males is usually a combination of symptoms and testosterone levels below either 350 or 230 ng/dl [39]. However, calculated free testosterone appears to be much more accurate in predicting clinically relevant issues or complications [40]. There is growing evidence that having higher FT levels predict favorably on the risk of low pathologic Gleason grade and faster recovery of sexual function (Fig. 4.8) [41]. In our

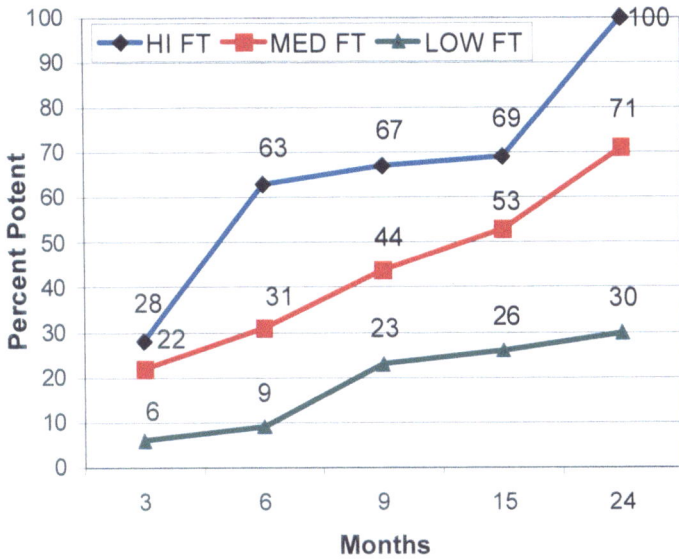

Fig. 4.8 Potency of patients in the authors series with follow-up of 24 months stratified by low (*green*), intermediate (*red*), and high (*blue*) serum-free testosterone levels following nerve-sparing robotic radical prostatectomy

opinion testosterone levels should be checked pre and postoperatively and if free levels are low men should have a discussion regarding replacement.

Postoperative Prophylaxis for Erectile Dysfunction

In experimental models it has been shown that injury to cavernous nerves in rats leads to endothelial cell apoptosis, decreased nitric oxide levels, and hypoxia leading to fibrosis and loss of smooth muscle in the corpora cavernosa [42–45]. In humans, there is clear evidence that fibrosis and loss of smooth muscle occurs and that vasculogenic effects occur as a result. Mulhall and associates first noted that arterial insufficiency occurs in approximately 50 % of patients following RP and does not improve within a year of surgery. In addition, approximately 50 % of patients developed venous leak 1 year following surgery which was also associated with a decreased return of erectile function [46]. Montorsi and associates reported that 6 months following surgery spontaneous erection occurred in 67% of patients who performed self-injection with PGE-1 compared to 20 % in patients that did not use injection therapy. Only 17 % of patients who injected PGE-1 developed venous leak by Doppler ultrasound criteria versus 53 % of patients who did not [47]. Similar findings have been reported both for PGE-1 urethral suppositories [48] (Alprostadil, Vivus) and vacuum devices [49].

In 2003 Padma-Nathan and associates in a randomized prospective study reported that 27 % of 51 patients who were potent prior to bilateral nerve-sparing radical retropubic prostatectomy who took sildenafil at bedtime for 9 months regained "full" potency versus only 4 % of patients that did not [50, 51]. These findings may possibly be explained by Schwartz and associates who examined the effect of sildenafil on the smooth muscle content of the corporal bodies after RRP. In this study, patients were divided into two groups: one receiving 50 mg every other night for 6 months following surgery and the other 100 mg. The higher dose group had a statistically significant increase in smooth muscle present on postoperative biopsy [52]. In similar fashion, Montorsi and colleagues in 2014 also confirmed an advantage to men who prophylactically took tadalafil in a randomized trial [53].

Although the cumulative knowledge regarding novel prophylactic treatments to hasten the return of erectile function in men following RRP is encouraging, there is no regimen that is clearly superior. Further, there is no consensus among experts with regard to the most effective agent or combination of agents to use. We currently recommend 5 mg of tadalafil nightly starting on the first postoperative day for all patients. For those patients who are highly motivated, PGE-1 self-injection three times per week is also offered.

References

1. Walsh PC, Donker PJ. Impotence following radical prostatectomy: insight into etiology and prevention. J Urol. 1982;128(3):492–7.
2. Walsh PC, Lepor H, Eggleston JC. Radical prostatectomy with preservation of sexual function: anatomical and pathological considerations. Prostate. 1983;4(5):473–85.
3. Seddon HJ, Medawar PB, Smith H. Rate of regeneration of peripheral nerves in man. J Physiol. 1943;102(2):191–215.
4. Rosen RC, Cappelleri JC, Smith MD, Lipsky J, Pena BM. Development and evaluation of an abridged, 5-item version of the International Index of Erectile Function (IIEF-5) as a diagnostic tool for erectile dysfunction. Int J Impot Res. 1999;11(6):319–26.
5. Parsons JK, Marschke P, Maples P, Walsh PC. Effect of methylprednisolone on return of sexual function after nerve-sparing radical retropubic prostatectomy. Urology. 2004;64(5):987–90.
6. Hara I, Kawabata G, Miyake H, Nakamura I, Hara S, Okada H et al. Comparison of quality of life following laparoscopic and open prostatectomy for prostate cancer. J Urol. 2003;169(6):2045–8.
7. Schover LR, Fouladi RT, Warneke CL, Neese L, Klein EA, Zippe C et al. Defining sexual outcomes after treatment for localized prostate carcinoma. Cancer. 2002;95(8):1773–85.
8. Rodriguez Jr E, Finley DS, Skarecky D, Ahlering TE. Single institution 2-year patient reported validated sexual function outcomes after nerve sparing robot assisted radical prostatectomy. J Urol. 2009;181(1):259–63.
9. Takenaka A, Murakami G, Matsubara A, Han SH, Fujisawa M. Variation in course of cavernous nerve with special reference to details of topographic relationships near prostatic apex: histologic study using male cadavers. Urology. 2005;65(1):136–42.
10. Takenaka A, Murakami G, Soga H, Jan SH, Arai Y, Fujisawa M. Anatomical analysis of the neurovascular bundle supplying penile cavernous tissue to ensure a reliable nerve graft after radical prostatectomy. J Urol. 2004;172(3):1032–5.
11. Takenaka A, Kawada M, Murakami G, Hisasue S, Tsukamoto T, Fujisawa M. Interindividual variation in distribution of extramural ganglion cells in the male pelvis: a semi-quantitative and immunohistochemical study concerning nerve-sparing pelvic surgery. Eur Urol. 2005;48(1):46–52. discussion 52.
12. Dorland's medical dictionary 25th ed, p. 1534.

13. Alsaid B, Karam I, Bessede T, Abdlsamad I, Uhl JF, Delmas V et al. Tridimensional computer-assisted anatomic dissection of posterolateral prostatic neurovascular bundles. Eur Urol. 2010;58(2):281–7.
14. Tewari A, Peabody JO, Fischer, Sarle R, Vallancien G, Delmas V et al. An operative and anatomic study to help in nerve sparing during laparoscopic and robotic radical prostatectomy. Eur Urol. 2003;43(5):444–54.
15. Tewari A, El-Hakim A, Horninger W, Peschel R, coll D, Bartsch G. Nerve-sparing during robotic radical prostatectomy: use of computer modeling and anatomic data to establish critical steps and maneuvers. Curr Urol Rep. 2005;6(2):126–8.
16. Costello AJ, Brooks M, Cole OJ. Anatomical studies of the neurovascular bundle and cavernosal nerves. BJU Int. 2004;94(7):1071–6.
17. Ganzer R, Stolzenburg JU, Wieland WF, Brundl J. Anatomic study of periprostatic nerve distribution: immunohistochemical differentiation of parasympathetic and sympathetic nerve fibres. Eur Urol. 2012;62(6):1150–6.
18. Hall-Craggs ECB. Anatomy as a basis for clinical medicine. Munchen: Urban and Schwarzenberg; 1990.
19. Schaumburg HH, Zotova E, Cannella B, Raine CS, Arezzo J, Tar M et al. Structural and functional investigations of the murine cavernosal nerve: a model system for serial spatio-temporal study of autonomic neuropathy. BJU Int. 2007;99(4):916–24.
20. Donoff BR. Nerve regeneration: basic and applied aspects. Cirt Rev Oral Biol Med. 1995;6(1):18–24.
21. Bray GM, Aguayo AJ. Regeneration of peripheral unmyelinated nerves. Fate of the axonal sprouts which develop after injury. J Anat. 1974;117(Pt 3):517–29.
22. Ahlering TE, Eichel L, Skarecky D. Rapid communication: early potency outcomes with cautery-free neurovascular bundle preservation with robotic laparoscopic radical prostatectomy. J Endourol. 2005;19(6):715–8.
23. Ahlering TE, Eichel L, Chou D, Skarecky DW. Feasibility study for robotic radical prostatectomy cautery-free neurovascular bundle preservation. Urology. 2005;65(5):994–7.
24. Ahlering TE, Skarecky D, Borin J. Impact of cautery versus cautery-free preservation of neurovascular bundles on early return of potency. J Endourol. 2006;20(8):586–9.
25. Ahlering TE, Eichel L, Skarecky D. Evaluation of long-term thermal injury using cautery during nerve sparing robotic prostatectomy. Urology. 2008;72(6):1371–4.
26. Wondergem J, Haveman J, Rusman V, Sminia P, Van Dijk JD. Effects of local hyperthermia on the motor function of the rat sciatic nerve. Int J Radiat Biol Relat Stud Phys Chem Med. 1988;53(3):429–38.
27. Hoogeveen JF, Troost D, Wondergem J, van der Kracht AH, Haveman J. Hyperthermic injury versus crush injury in the rat sciatic nerve: a comparative functional, histopathological and morphometrical study. J Neurol Sci. 1992;108(1):55–64.
28. Donzelli J, Leonetti JP, Wurster RD, Lee JM, Young MR. Neuroprotection due to irrigation during bipolar cautery. Arch Otolaryngol Head Neck Surg. 2000;126(2):149–53.
29. Ong AM, Su LM, Varkarakis I, Inagaki T, Link RE, Bhayani SB et al. Nerve sparing radical prostatectomy: effects of hemostatic energy sources on the recovery of cavernous nerve function in a canine model. J Urol. 2004;172(4 Pt 1):1318–22.
30. Mandhani A, Dorsey PJ Jr., Ramanatha R, Salamanca JI, Rao S, Leung R et al. Real time monitoring of temperature changes in neurovascular bundles during robotic radical prostatectomy: thermal map for nerve-sparing radical prostatectomy. J Endourol. 2008;22(10):2313–7.
31. Khan F, Rodriquez E, Finley DS, Skarecky DW, Ahlering TE. Spread of thermal energy and heat sinks: implications for nerve-sparing robotic prostatectomy. J Endourol. 2007;21(10):1195–8.
32. Zorn KC, Bhojani N, Gautam G, Shikanov S, Gofrit ON, Jayram G et al. Application of ice cold irrigation during vascular pedicle control of robot-assisted radical prostatectomy: EnSeal instrument cooling to reduce collateral thermal tissue damage. J Endourol. 2010;24(12):1991–6.
33. Kowalczyk KJ, Huang AC, Hevelone ND, Lipsitz SR, Yu HY, Ulmer WD et al. Stepwise approach for nerve sparing without countertraction during robot-assisted radical prostatectomy: technique and outcomes. Eur Urol. 2011;60(3):536–47.

34. Montorsi F, Wilson TG, Rosen RC, Ahlering TE, Artibani W, Carroll PR et al. Best practices in robot-assisted radical prostatectomy: recommendations of the Pasadena Consensus Panel. Eur Urol. 2012;62(3):368–81.
35. Finley DS, Rodriguez E Jr., Skarecky DW, Ahlering TE. Quantitative and qualitative analysis of the recovery of potency after radical prostatectomy: effect of unilateral vs bilateral nerve sparing. BJU Int. 2009;104(10):1484–9.
36. Walsh PC, Epstein JI, Lowe FC. Potency following radical prostatectomy with wide unilateral excision of the neurovascular bundle. J Urol. 1987;138(4):823–7.
37. Kundu SD, Roehl KA, Eggener SE, Antenor JA, Han M, Catalona WJ. Potency, continence and complications in 3,477 consecutive radical retropubic prostatectomies. J Urol. 2004;172(6 Pt 1):2227–31.
38. Traish AM, Saad F, Feeley RJ, Guay A. The dark side of testosterone deficiency: III. Cardiovascular disease. J Androl. 2009;30(5):477–94.
39. Morales A. Andorgen deficiency in the aging male. In: Wein K et al., editors. Campbell-Walsh urology, Vol 1. 10th ed. Philadelphia, PA: Elsevier; 2012.
40. Ahlering TE, Morales B, Chang A, Skarecky D. Low free testosterone (FT) versus total testos-terone (TT) in predicting potency following robotic-assisted radical prostatectomy. J Endourol. 2010;24(Suppl):A46, PS 6–24.
41. Ahlering TE, Morales B, Lusch A, Skarecky D. For preoperatively potent men free testoster-one levels are predictive of time to potency following robotic-assisted radical prostatectomy. J Endourol. 2012;26(Suppl):A81–2.
42. Klein LT, Miller MI, Buttyan R, Raffo AJ, Burchard M, Devris G et al. Apoptosis in the rat penis after penile denervation. J Urol. 1997;158(2):626–30.
43. Rehman J, Ghrist GJ, Kaynan A, Samadi D, Fleischmann J. Intraoperative electrical stimula-tion of cavernosal nerves with monitoring of intracorporeal pressure in patients undergoing nerve sparing radical prostatectomy. BJU Int. 1999;84(3):305–10.
44. User HM, Hairston JH, Zelner DJ, McKenna KE, McVary KT. Penile weight and cell subtype specific changes in a post-radical prostatectomy model of erectile dysfunction. J Urol. 2003;169(3):1175–9.
45. Leungwattanakij S, Bivalacqua TJ, Usta MF, Yang DY, Hyun JS, Champion HC et al. Cavernous neurotomy causes hypoxia and fibrosis in rat corpus cavernosum. J Androl. 2003;24(2):239–45.
46. Mulhall JP, Slovick R, Hotaling J, Aviv N, Valenzuela R, Waters WB. Erectile dysfunction after radical prostatectomy: hemodynamic profiles and their correlation with the recovery of erectile function. J Urol. 2002;167(3):1371–5.
47. Montorsi F, Guazzoni G, Strambi LF, DaPozzo LF, Nava L, Barbieri L. Recovery of spontane-ous erectile function after nerve-sparing radical retropubic prostatectomy with and without early intracavernous injections of alprostadil: results of a prospective, randomized trial. J Urol. 1997;158(4):1408–10.
48. Zippe C. Early use of MUSE following radical prostatectomy facilitates earlier return of erectile function and successful sexual activity. Irvine, CA: A.R.T. Symposium, Editor; 2006.
49. Raina R, Agarwal A, Ausmundson S, Lakin M, Nandipati KC, Montague DK et al. Early use of vacuum constriction device following radical prostatectomy facilitates early sexual activity and potentially earlier return of erectile function. Int J Impot Res. 2006;18(1):77–81.
50. Padma-Nathan H et al. Postoperative nightly administration of sildenafil citrate significanty improves the return of normal spontaneous erectile function after bilateral nerve sparing radical prostatectomy. J Urol. 2003;169(Suppl):1402.
51. Padma-Nathan H, McCullough A, Forest C. Erectile dysfunction secondary to nerve-sparing radical retropubic prostatectomy: comparative phosphodiesterase-5 inhibitor efficacy for ther-apy and novel prevention strategies. Curr Urol Rep. 2004;5(6):467–71.
52. Schwartz EJ, Wong P, Graydon RJ. Sildenafil preserves intracorporeal smooth muscle after radical retropubic prostatectomy. J Urol. 2004;171(2 Pt 1):771–4.
53. Montorsi F, Brock G, Stolzenburg JU, Mulhall J, Moncada I, Patel HR et al. Effects of Tadalafil treatment on erectile function recovery following bilateral nerve-sparing radical prostatec-tomy: A randomized placebo-controlled study (REACTT). Eur Urol. 2014;65:587–96.

Chapter 5
Technical Innovations to Optimize Early Return of Urinary Continence

Usama Khater and Sanjay Razdan

Introduction

Post-prostatectomy incontinence (PPI) represents a time-dependent devastating iatrogenic complication after surgery. A 12-month continence rate is reported in 48–91 % after laparoscopic prostatectomy (LP), in 89–97 % after robot-assisted laparoscopic prostatectomy (RALP) and 77.7–93.7 % of cases after open retropubic radical prostatectomy (RRP) [1]. Although the continence rate 1 year after RALP is excellent, achievement of an earlier continence at 3 and 6 months postoperatively is still a challenge. Several surgical techniques to optimize the early return of continence have been described. Most of these techniques emphasize the importance of restoring the normal pelvic anatomy after removal of the prostate.

Anatomical Background and Techniques

In men, urinary continence is thought to be controlled by five main structures: the detrusor muscle, the internal sphincter, the ureterotrigonal muscles, the levator muscles, and the rhabdosphincter [2, 3]. Maintaining these structures and maintaining

Electronic supplementary material The online version of this chapter (doi:10.1007/978-3-319-39448-0_5) contains supplementary material, which is available to authorized users.

U. Khater, M.D. • S. Razdan, M.D., M.Ch. (✉)
International Robotic Prostatectomy Institute, Urology Center of Excellence at Jackson South Hospital, Deering Medical Plaza, 9380 SW 150th Street, Suite 200, Miami, FL 33176, USA
e-mail: sanjayrazdanmd@gmail.com

the normal anatomy of the pelvis are the cornerstone to achieve better post-RALP results. This can be achieved through three different steps of techniques: preservation, reconstruction, and reinforcement of the sphincter structures.

Preservation

Bladder Neck Preservation

Anatomically, the bladder neck serves as an internal sphincter and it is intuitive that bladder neck preservation may contribute to early return of urinary continence.

Maintaining circular fibers of the bladder neck during dissection of the prostato-vesical junction can accelerate the return of postoperative urinary continence. Anterocephalic tension of the bladder using the fourth arm will create a landmark that facilitates dissection of the bladder neck. Precise incision of the posterior bladder neck will maintain clean detrusor margins for subsequent urethrovesical anastomosis, Figs. 5.1, 5.2, and 5.3 [4].

Friedlander et al. compared cancer control outcomes and continence in bladder neck sparing vs. non sparing technique during RALP. No difference in cancer control outcome was detected in both groups. However, bladder neck sparing is associated with fewer urinary leakage complication and better post-prostatectomy continence outcome [4].

Nerve Preservation

The rhabdosphincter receives nerve fibers from the pelvic nerve, intrapelvic branch and perineal branch from pudendal nerve. Preservation of intrapelvic branch of the pudendal nerve has been shown to maintain rhabdosphincter function after RALP [5].

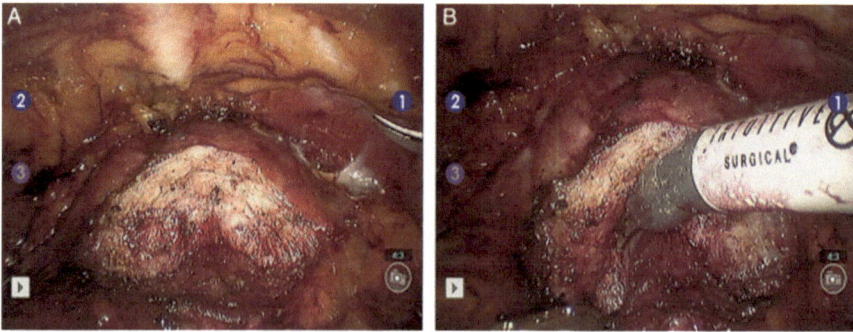

Fig. 5.1 Bladder neck dissection is initiated in midline at prostate mid/base anterior until reaching depth of vertically oriented bladder neck fibers (**a**). Bladder neck incision is arced cephalad with lateral extension until anterior portion of bladder neck is defined. Blunt dissection is performed anterior, and on right and left (**b**) of bladder neck to define its funneled contour as it transitions to prostatic urethra [4]

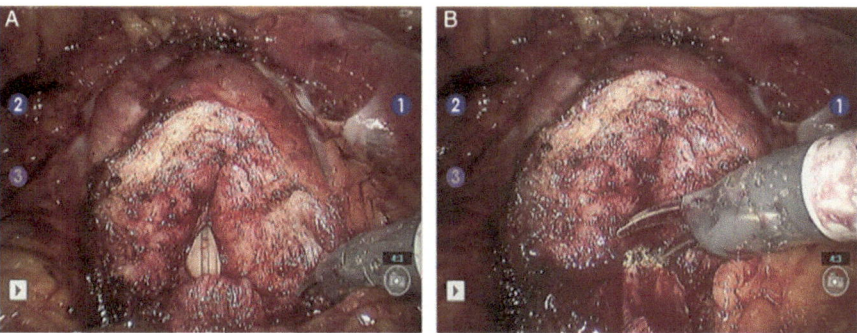

Fig. 5.2 Bladder neck is opened anterior to expose catheter (**a**), which is withdrawn before scoring posterior bladder neck mucosa with monopolar current (**b**) [4]

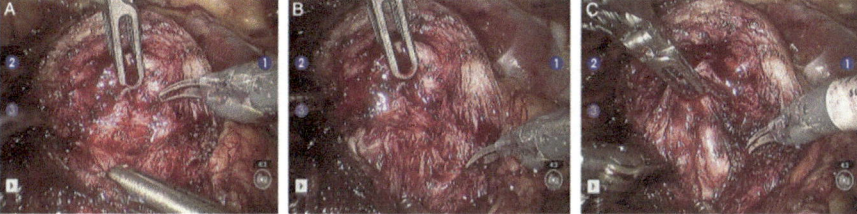

Fig. 5.3 Fourth arm ProGrasp elevates prostate base to create tension for posterior bladder neck dissection (**a**). Assistant laparoscopic grasper counter traction is applied during posterior bladder neck dissection. Bladder neck dissection proceeds laterally to adipose tissue, which serves as lateral border of dissection bilaterally (**b**). Downward traction of assistant suction tip aids exposure. Note suction tip on posterior longitudinal detrusor layer. Posterior longitudinal detrusor layer is opened as low as possible, revealing vas deferens (**c**) [4]

Though it is clear that neurovascular bundle preservation during RALP will preserve postoperative potency, it is still controversial whether preservation of nerves around the bladder, prostate, and urethra results in continence after RALP. Choi et al. reported that continence rate and EPIC urinary function score were better for bilateral nerve-sparing vs. non-nerve-sparing technique after 4 months [6]. On the other hand, Pick et al. have found no significant difference in continence rate at 12 months after RALP between unilateral, bilateral, and non-nerve-sparing RALP (88.9, 89.2, and 84.8 % respectively), concluding that preservation of cavernous nerve does not predict over all return of continence [7].

Pubovesical Complex Sparing and Puboprostatic Ligament Preservation

Different studies have shown that puboprostatic ligament preservation improves continence results after RALP [8, 9]. Astimakopoulos et al. developed a pubovesical complex sparing technique, in which the prostate is dissected from underneath the spared pubovesical complex and urethrovesical anastomosis is performed under the spared complex. Twenty percent of patients needed one security pad after catheter removal. Preservation of periprostatic anatomy may enhance early functional outcome [10].

Preservation of Urethral Length

Male sphincteric mechanism is composed of striated urogenital sphincter muscle and an inner smooth muscle layer. The internal component of the distal sphincter mechanism extends to the verumontanum while the striated sphincter is functional from prostate apex to the bulb [11]. Early urinary continence can be achieved through maximum preservation of the striated sphincter and intraprostatic portion of the membranous urethra [12]. It is important not to compromise apical margin during maximal urethral length preservation, this can be achieved by accurate identification of the junction between prostatic apex and urethra. Nguyen et al. stated that shorter urethral sphincter length on pre operative endorectal MRI is associated with higher risk of post-prostatectomy incontinence. However, technical modification to restore the continence mechanism intraoperatively could improve continence outcome in patients with shorter urethral sphincter [13].

Modified Maximal Urethral Length Preservation (MULP) Technique

At the International Robotic Prostatectomy Institute, the senior author and editor of this text (*Razdan S*) modified and pioneered maximal urethral length preservation (MULP) in RALP. In this technique the previously ligated deep venous complex (DVC) is divided using shears. The correct plane between the anterior prostatic capsule and the ligated DVC is achieved by the "apical pinch" which affords proper orientation as well as avoids a positive anterior margin. Following division of the deep venous complex, the apex is dissected carefully along the retropubic plane using the robotic endoshear, starting at the prostatic–rhabdosphincter junction, by dividing the striated and smooth muscle fibers sweeping from the apex toward the membranous urethra. Twisting the prostate from side to side with the fourth robot arm enables clear visualization of the prostatic apex. Subsequently, division of the flimsy posterior fibrous connections at the apex of the prostate allows release of the posterior lip of the prostate, thereby exposing an additional length of intraprostatic urethra, which adds to the MULP (Fig. 5.4). Division of the urethra at the new prostate urethral junction is then carried out with a birds eye view thereby, reducing positive apical margins (see Video 5.1). The authors have been able to preserve an additional 1–2 cm of intraprostatic and membranous urethra by this modified MULP procedure which in turn facilitates an easier vesicourethral anastomosis and earlier return of continence. Urethrovesical anastomosis is then performed using the classic Van Velthoven technique (see Video 5.2).

The continence rate following the modified MULP technique in RALP was in 50–70 % of patients at one month, in 90–96.66 % at 3 months and 100 % of patients 6 months after catheter removal [14].

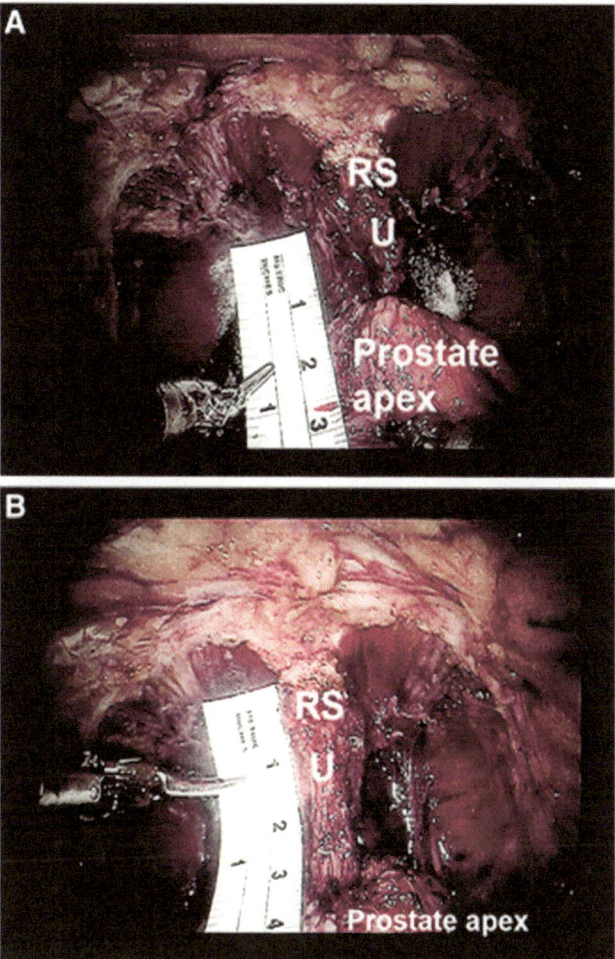

Fig. 5.4 (**a**) The posterior urethral junction and the membranous urethra after dissecting the endo-pelvic fascia and the dorsal vein complex. (**b**) The maximal urethral length preservation after performing the retro-apical dissection. *RS* rhabdosphincter, *U* membranous urethra [14]

A considerable proportion of the external urethral sphincter is located between the verumontanum and distal edge of the prostatic apex, and this plays a significant role in continence. Through MULP technique we were able to get an extra length of urethral stump that improved the overall continence mechanism. The longer urethral stump also facilitates faster and easily accessible vesicourethral anastomosis without the need for perineal compression and provides support to the bladder. By dissecting the urethra more proximally in MULP, we keep the autonomic branches that innervate the external sphincter away from the anastomosis. Furthermore, by working more proximally away from the external sphincter, the latter is less likely to be compromised by the inflammatory process that takes place due to intraoperative maneuvers at the site of the anastomosis. Other studies have also reiterated that MULP has a very significant role in early continence recovery [15].

Reconstruction

Posterior Rhabdosphincter Reconstruction

Posterior reconstruction aims at restoring the anatomical and functional defect through reapproximating the posterior semi-circumference of the rhabdosphincter to the residual cut edge of the Denonvilliers' fascia. This will allow a firm support to the posterior aspect of the urethral sphincter complex [16–18]. Nguyen et al. investigated the relation between posterior reconstruction and early return of continence after RALP and LRP, 3 days after catheter removal, 34 % of patients who underwent posterior reconstruction were continent, in comparison to patients who underwent standard technique where only 3 % were continent ($P=0.007$) [19]. Brien et al. have reported a significant improvement in terms of return of baseline score for urinary bother in posterior reconstruction group in comparison to control group (72 % vs. 53 %; $P=0.0083$) [20]. Gondo et al. have reported that posterior reconstruction has better early recovery of urinary continence results after 1 month of catheter removal in univariate analysis [21]. Fecarra et al. have reported 95 % recovery of urinary continence at a mean follow-up of 9 months [22] He also concluded that posterior reconstruction procedure is simple, with minimal increase in operative time, and provides a good support of the urethrovesical anastomosis. On the other hand, Menon et al. have found no significant difference in continence rate with posterior reconstruction compared to control group [23].

Anterior Retropubic Suspension

Anterior retropubic suspension aims at providing anatomical support of the urethra and stabilizing urethra and striated sphincter in anatomical position [24]. Anterior suspension is done through a monofilament suture that pass from the right to the left between the urethra and dorsal venous complex and then through the periosteum of the pubic bone. Patel et al. have reported significant improvement in continence rate after 3 months of RALP, in patients who had anterior suspension technique in comparison to non suspension technique (92.8 % vs. 83 %, $P=0.02$) [25].

At our institution we compared the continence rates at 1, 3, and 6 months after RALP in three group of patients; the first group had posterior urethral reconstruction and anterior bladder suspension, second group had MULP combined with posterior urethral reconstruction and anterior bladder suspension and the third group had only MULP. Each group included 30 matched patients. The second and third groups showed significantly higher and earlier continence rate than the first group who had posterior urethral reconstruction and anterior bladder suspension without

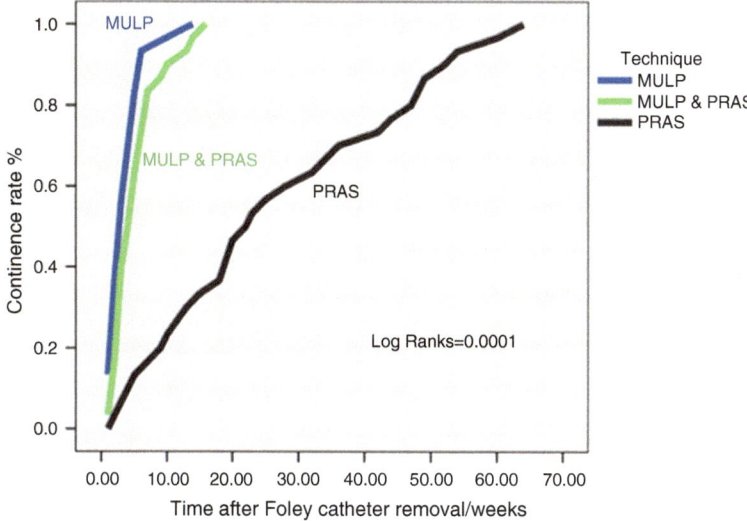

Fig. 5.5 Kaplan–Meier plot for the improvement in continence rates among the three study groups. *MULP* maximal urethral length preservation, *PRAS* posterior urethral reconstruction and anterior bladder suspension

MULP. There was no significant difference in the continence rate between the patients who had only MULP and the group who had MULP combined with posterior urethral reconstruction and anterior bladder suspension, Fig. 5.5. No significant differences were noticed in the rates of overall and apical positive margins between the three groups. No significant variations were detected in terms of biochemical recurrence at 12 month follow-up [14].

Total Reconstruction of Vesicourethral Junction

Tewari et al. evaluated continence rate in patients who underwent anterior reconstruction alone versus anterior and posterior reconstruction during RALP versus a historical control group, he found that at 3 months, the continence rate for the control group was 50 %, while in the anterior reconstruction group and combined anterior and posterior reconstruction groups continence rate was 77 and 91 % respectively at 3 months [15]. A much more reconstruction techniques were used including: Preservation of archus tendentious and puboprostatic ligament, creation of muscular flap behind the sphincter, control of dorsal venous complex using a puboprostatic ligament sparing suture, preparation of a long urethral sump, usage of Pagano principle reinforcement of the flap behind the bladder neck, usage of Rocco principle suturing of the flap to the distal end of the Denonvillier's fascia close to the urethral stump. Finally, reattachment of Arcus tendentious and puboprostatic plate to the bladder neck after the anastomosis is created [2] (Fig. 5.6).

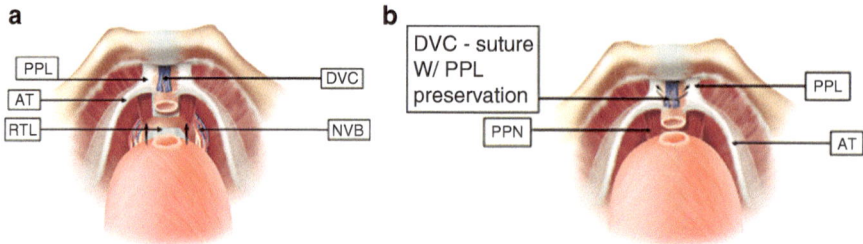

Fig. 5.6 (**a**) Creation of muscle flap behind the bladder. (**b**) Control of dorsal venous complex using a puboprostatic ligament sparing suture [15]. *PPL* puboprostatic ligament, *NVB* neurovascular bundle. *AT* arcus tendentious, *DVC* deep venous complex, *RTLL* retroperitoneal layer

Reinforcement

Bladder Neck Plication

Bladder neck plication is done through a plication stitch placed 2 cm proximal to the vesicourethral anastomosis at 3 o'clock and 9 o'clock, after tying this stitch, this will create a funneling of distal bladder neck. Mean time to total continence was 35.10 ± 3.8 weeks in stitch technique group, vs. 8.49 ± 6.32 weeks in non stitch group ($P=0.002$) [26].

Bladder Neck Sling Suspension

Bladder neck sling suspension can support proximal urethra and bladder neck and increase the functional length of the urethral sphincteric complex after RALP. This subsequently improves the early return of continence after RALP [27].

Conclusions

– Surgical modifications that preserve the natural urinary continence mechanisms seem to promote early recovery of continence.
– Maximal urethral length preservation (MULP) in the authors' experience is the single most important factor determining early return of continence after RALP.
– Neurovascular bundle preservation and bladder neck preservation may have a positive impact in overall recovery of urinary continence, though the results of studies are mixed.
– In the authors' experience, anterior suspension and total vesicourethral reconstruction have no impact on recovery of continence and in fact may have a detrimental effect on early return of continence.

References

1. Park B, Kim W, Jeong BC, et al. Comparison of oncological and functional outcomes of pure versus robotic assisted radical prostatectomy performed by a single surgeon. Scand J Urol. 2013;47:10–8.
2. Golomb J, Chertin B, Mor Y. Anatomy of urinary continence and neurogenic incontinence. Therapy. 2009;6:151–5.
3. Koraitim MM. The male urethral sphincter complex revisited: an anatomical concept and its physiological correlate. J Urol. 2008;179:1683–9.
4. Friedlander D, Alemozaffar M, Hevelon N, Lipsitz S, Hu J. Stepwise description and outcomes of bladder neck sparing during robot-assisted laparoscopic radical prostatectomy. J Urol. 2012;188:1754–60.
5. Hollabaugh R, Dmochwski R, Kneib T, Steiner M. Preservation of putative continence nerves during radical retropubic prostatectomy leads to more rapid return of urinary incontinence. Urology. 1998;51:960–7.
6. Choi W, Freire M, Soukup J, Lipsitz S, Carvas F, Williams S, et al. Nerve sparing technique and urinary control after robot assisted laparoscopic prostatectomy. World J Urol. 2011;29:21–7.
7. Pick D, Osann K, Skarecky D, Narula N, Finley D, Ahlering T. The impact of cavernous nerve preservation on continence after robotic radical prostatectomy. BJU Int. 2011;108:1492–6.
8. Avant O, Jones J, Beck H, Hunt C, Staub M. New method to improve treatment outcomes after radical prostatectomy. Urology. 2000;56:658–62.
9. Stolzenburg J, Liastsikos E, Rabenalt R, Do M, Sakelaropoulos G, Horn L, et al. Nerve sparing endoscopic extraperitoneal radical prostatectomy – effect of puboprostatic ligament preservation on early continence and positive margins. Eur Urol. 2006;49:103–11.
10. Asimakopoulos A, Annino F, D'Orazio A, Pereira R. Complete periprostatic anatomy preservation during robotic assisted laparoscopic radical prostatectomy (RALP): the new pubovesical complex sparing technique. Eur Urol. 2010;58:407–17.
11. Hakimi A, Faleck D, Agalliu I, Rozenblit A, Chrnyak V, Ghavaamian R. Preoperative and intraoperative measurements of urethral length as predictors of continence after robotic assisted radical prostatectomy. J Endourol. 2011;25:1025–30.
12. Van Randenborgh H, Paul R, Kubler H, Breul J, Hartung R. Improved urinary continence after radical prostatectomy with preparation of a long partially portion of the membranous urethra: analysis of 1013 consecutive cases. Prostate Cancer Prostatic Dis. 2004;7:253–7.
13. Nguyen L, Jhaveri J, Twari A. Surgical technique to overcome anatomical shortcoming: balancing post-prostatectomy continence outcomes of urethral sphincter lengths on preoperative magnetic resonance imaging. J Urol. 2008;179:1907–11.
14. Hamada A, Razdan S, Etafy M, Fagin R, Razdan S. Early return of continence in patients undergoing robot assisted laparoscopic prostatectomy using modified maximal urethral length preservation technique. J Endourol. 2014;28:930–8.
15. Tewari A, Jhaveri J, Rao S, Yadav R, Bartsch G, Te A, et al. Total reconstruction of vesicourethral junction. BJU Int. 2008;101:871–7.
16. Rocco F, Rocco B. Anatomical reconstruction of the rhabdosphincter after radical prostatectomy. BJU Int. 2009;104:274–81.
17. Rocco F, Carmignan L, Acquati P, Gadda F, Dell'Orto P, Rocco B, et al. Restoration of posterior aspect of rhabdosphincter shortens continence time after radical prostatectomy. J Urol. 2006;175:2201–6.
18. Rocco F, Carmignani L, Acquati P, Gadda F, Dell'Orto P, Rocco B, et al. Early continence recovery after open radical prostatectomy with restoration of the posterior aspect of the rhabdosphincter. Eur Urol. 2007;52:376–83.
19. Nguyen M, Kamoi K, Stein R, Aron M, Hafron J, Turna B, et al. Early continence outcomes of posterior musculofascial plate reconstruction during robotic and laparoscopic prostatectomy. BJU Int. 2008;101:1135–9.

20. Brien J, Barone B, Fabrizio M, Given R. Posterior reconstruction before vesicourethral anastomosis in patients undergoing robot assisted laparoscopic prostatectomy leads to earlier return to baseline continence. J Endourol. 2011;25:441–5.
21. Gondo T, Yoshika K, Hashimoto T, Nakagami Y, Hamada R, Kashima T, et al. The powerful impact of double-layered posterior rhabdosphincter reconstruction on early recovery of urinary continence after robot assisted radical prostatectomy. J Endourol. 2012;26:1159–64.
22. Ficarra V, Gan M, Borghesi M, Zattoni F, Mottrie A. Posterior muscolofascial reconstruction incorporated into urethrovesical anastomosis during robot assisted radical prostatectomy. J Endourol. 2012;26:1542–5.
23. Menon M, Muhletaler F, Campos M, Peabody J. Assessment of early continence after reconstruction of periprostatic tissues in patient undergoing computer assisted (robotic) prostatectomy: results of a 2 groups parallel randomized controlled trial. J Urol. 2008;180:1018–23.
24. Hurtes X, Rouret M, Vaessen C, Perreira H, Faiver d'Arcier B, Cormier L, et al. Anterior suspension combined with posterior reconstruction during robot assisted laparoscopic prostatectomy improves early return of urinary incontinence: a prospective randomized multicenter trial. BJU Int. 2012;110:875–83.
25. Patel V, Coelho R, Palmer K, Rocco B. Periurethral suspension stitch during robot assisted laparoscopic radical prostatectomy: description of the technique and continence outcomes. Eur Urol. 2009;56:472–8.
26. Lee D, Wedmid A, Mendoza P, Sharma S, Walicki M, Hastings R, et al. Bladder neck Plication stitch: a novel technique during robot assisted radical prostatectomy to improve recovery of urinary incontinence. J Endourol. 2011;25:1873–7.
27. Kojima Y, Hamakawa T, Kubota Y, Ogawa S, Haga N, Tozawa K, et al. Bladder neck sling suspension during robot assisted radical prostatectomy to improve early return of urinary continence: a comparative analysis. Urology. 2014;83:632–9.

Chapter 6
Technical Innovations to Optimize Early Return of Erectile Function

Gabriel Ogaya-Pinies, Vladimir Mouraviev, Hariharan Ganapathi, and Vipul Patel

Introduction

With radical prostatectomy (RP) delivering better survival results, preservation of erectile function has become an increasing priority among patients who choose surgery as the first line of treatment. To date, the ideal outcome cannot be limited to oncologic freedom since contemporary patients, due to their young age, are motivated to preserve their sexual function and urinary continence.

Before the discovery of the neurovascular bundles (NVBs) by Walsh and Donker [1], the cause of erectile dysfunction following RP was not completely understood. Since the introduction of the anatomic nerve-sparing (NS) technique, the injury to the cavernous nerve intraoperatively may be preventable. An adequate surgical technique that minimizes the damage to the NVBs plays a key role in preservation and functional recovery.

Present day, the neurovascular preservation is accomplished by the surgeon's expertise and knowledge of the anatomy, as well as by the improvements of visualization, instrumentation, and magnification provided by novel robotic systems. In this chapter, we discuss fundamental aspects of the neurovascular anatomy, define landmarks and principles for a NS radical prostatectomy, and also review some of the new technological developments designed to help surgeons to perform these critical steps and achieve an early return of the erectile function.

G. Ogaya-Pinies (✉) • V. Mouraviev • H. Ganapathi • V. Patel
Global Robotics Institute, Florida Hospital-Celebration Health,
410 Celebration Place, Suite 200, Celebration, FL 34747, USA
e-mail: Gabriel.ogayapinies@flhosp.org

© Springer International Publishing Switzerland 2016
S. Razdan (ed.), *Urinary Continence and Sexual Function After Robotic Radical Prostatectomy*, DOI 10.1007/978-3-319-39448-0_6

83

Anatomy of Neurovascular Bundles

The pelvic splenic nerves arise from the anterior sacral roots, with most branches originating from S4 and smaller contribution of S2 and S3. These parasympathetic fibers converge with sympathetic fibers from the hypogastric nerve to form the pelvis plexus.

The inferior extension of the pelvic plexus unites with several vessels to form the neurovascular bundle (NVB) of Walsh. This tubular structure runs along the dorsolateral aspect of the prostate gland enclosed in fascial sheets and intimately associates with the capsular vessels of the prostate.

Many anatomic studies have suggested that in addition to the NVB, multiples accessory channels exist that ramify in the prostatic and Denonvillier's fascia and which supply neural stimulation of the penis. These accessory fibers, which form an apical plexus on the posterolateral aspect of the prostatic apex and urethra, could potentially act as a neural pathway for the urethral sphincter [2] (Fig. 6.1).

Prostatic Vasculature as a Landmark for Nerve-Sparing RARP

There is a lack of clear macroscopic landmarks to identify the NVB during a radical prostatectomy. We have identified intraoperative elements of the prostate vasculature as anatomical reference points, key to display natural separation planes between

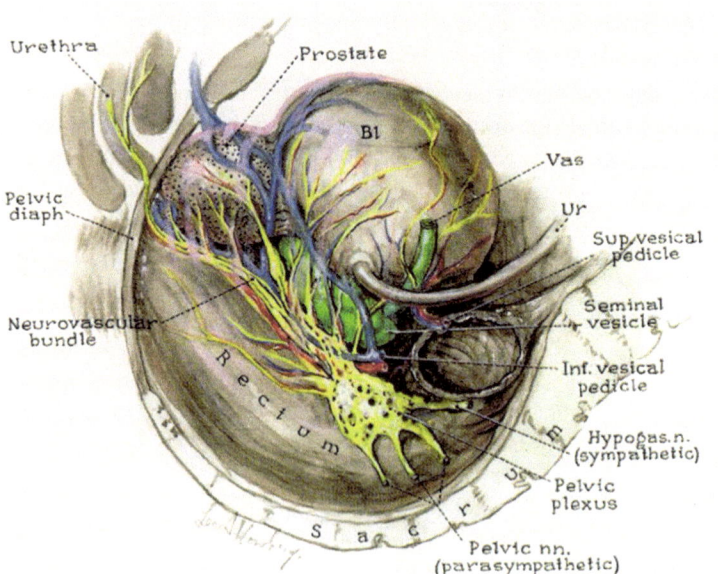

Fig. 6.1 Anatomy of the pelvic plexus and neurovascular bundles. Courtesy of J. Urol. 138:1402–1406, 1987

the prostate and the neurovascular bundle. This allows us to perform the nerve sparing in a more standardized and consistent manner. A landmark artery (LA) was identified running on the lateral border of the prostate corresponding to either a prostatic or capsular artery.

The arterial supply to the prostate originates from the internal iliac (or hypogastric) artery [3, 4]. The prostatic artery (PA) is a branch of the vesicoprostatic trunk and reaches the prostate on its anterolateral aspect at the base [5]. From there, it can continue distally down to the perineum or give origin to a network of capsular arteries (CAs) running along the lateral border of the prostate [6]. During their course alongside the prostate, these elements of the prostatic vasculature (PV), especially the CAs, are related intimately with the capsular nerve (CNs) and provide a scaffold to the nerves at their course along the prostate [7]. Therefore, the PV may provide a macroscopic landmark for identifying and preserving the CNs at the time of surgery.

After opening sharply the levator fascia over the prostate, the presence of a distinctive PA could be found posterior laterally between the midprostate and the base. The artery enters the prostate on the anterolateral aspect, and it is easily recognized by its large size and tortuosity (Fig. 6.2). Delicately developing a plane of dissection between the PA and the prostate results in a natural detachment of the NVB from the prostate. For a complete NS, the correct plane of dissection is recognized by the presence of pearly areolar tissue and is gently developed posteriorly following the prostatic contour until the previously created posterior plane is reached.

Another common finding is the absence of a distinctive PA and the presence of multiple CAs. These arteries are found on the lateral aspect of the prostate, forming a mesh throughout the thickness of the NVB. The most superficial of these CAs can be recognized after opening the levator fascia over the prostate. It is located over the medial border of the NVB fat, close to the point where the fat ends over the prostate (Fig. 6.3).

Nerve-sparing approach can be classified as either medial or lateral to the landmark artery. Fine tailoring on the medial border of the landmark artery can consis-

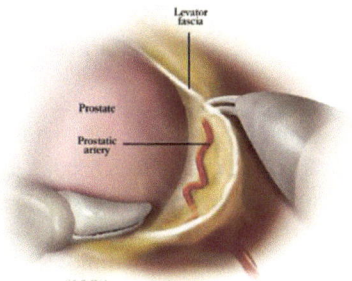 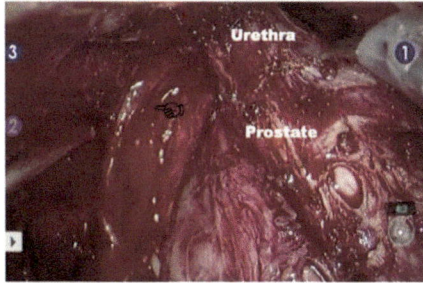

Fig. 6.2 *Left*: The prostatic artery (PA) can be recognized after opening the levator fascia on the base of the prostate. It has a large diameter and a tortuous configuration, which makes it easy to be recognized intraoperatively. It continues alongside the prostate occupying the medial aspect of the neurovascular bundle (NVB). *Right*: Complete left nerve sparing; the prostate has been detached from the NVB. Note how the pointed PA follows the course of the NVB and enters the perineum behind the urethra

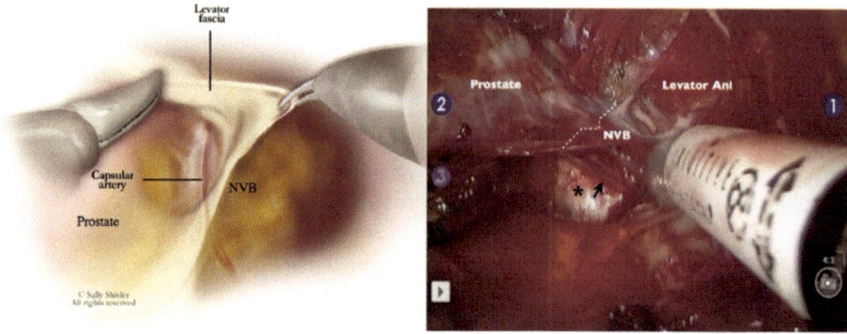

Fig. 6.3 *Left*: Capsular arteries (CAs) can be recognized after opening the levator fascia. They are found more distally than the prostatic artery (PA), at the level of the midprostate. CAs are thin, harder to identify, and do not have a tortuous configuration like the PA. They usually end in small twigs at the apex and do not perforate into the perineum. *Right*: A plane of dissection has been developed between the landmark CA and the prostate. Notice that as the dissection gets deeper, additional CAs are found along the medial aspect of the neurovascular bundle (NVB; *arrow*). The right plane of dissection for a complete nerve sparing is to stay on the medial aspect of the CAs, through the pearly areolar tissue between the prostate and the NVB (*asterisk*)

Table 6.1 Area of residual nerve tissue according with the technique of nerve-sparing procedure

Anatomical quantitative evaluation	Technique of nerve sparing in relation to prostatic artery		
	Medial	Lateral	p-Value
Area of residual nerve tissue	0 (0–3) mm²	14 (9–25) mm²	<0.001

tently result in a complete nerve sparing, whereas performing the nerve sparing on its lateral border results in several degrees of incomplete partial nerve sparing (Table 6.1).

Anatomic Grading of Nerve Sparing During RARP

The goal of NS during RP is to preserve the greatest possible amount of nerve tissue without compromising surgical margins. In this context, a very elegant manipulation is necessary to achieve the precise amount of nerve preservation needed for an individual patient. Schatloff et al. [8] described a standardized NS grading system based on intraoperative visual cues. The NS was graded by the surgeon intraoperatively before specimen extraction independently for either side as follows: 1=no NS; 2=<50 NS; 3=50 % NS; 4=75 % NS; 5=95 % NS. The technique consisted of sharp opening the levator fascia and identification of the LA with its course in retrograde manner up to the pedicle. This way, we were able to show a significant correlation between a higher NSS and a decreased area of residual nerve tissue on prostatectomy specimens (Fig. 6.4).

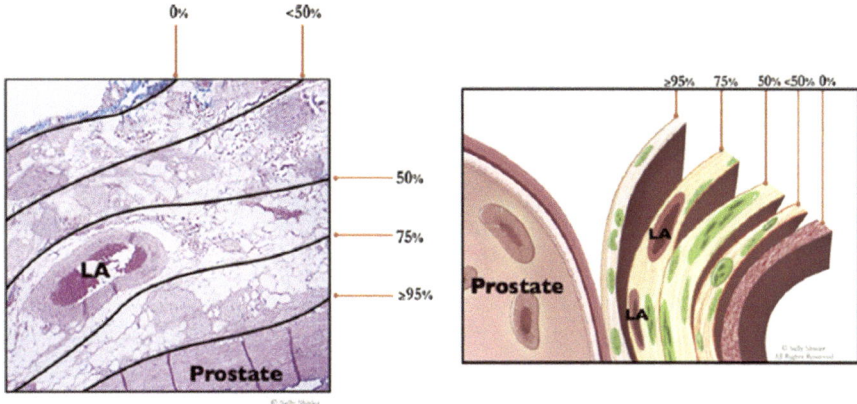

Fig. 6.4 A cross-section of the neurovascular bundle, represented as a histology slide (*left*) and a didactic diagram (*right*), demonstrates our graded approach to nerve sparing (NS). Several degrees of partial NS can be obtained when paying careful attention to the anatomic cues that are discussed. *LA* landmark artery

In our recently updated series of 2036 patients, the potency outcomes suggested that our subjective NS system predicted potency recovery and indicated that even minor nerve trauma significantly prolonged EF recovery. By Kaplan–Meier analysis, recovery of potency is more rapid in higher NS grades (grade 2 vs. grade 3, log-rank $p = 0.032$; grade 3 vs. grade 4, log-rank $p < 0.001$; grade 4 vs. grade 5, log-rank $p < 0.001$) (Fig. 6.5).

Key Principles of Neurovascular Preservation

The goal of nerve sparing during RARP is to preserve the greatest possible amount of nerve tissue without compromising surgical margins. A very meticulous approach is necessary to achieve the precise amount of nerve preservation needed for an individual patient. In our institution, we established our approach to avoid an excessive traction, use of thermal energy, or direct damage during dissection (Fig. 6.6).

Retrograde Versus Antegrade Nerve Sparing During RARP

Techniques to preserve the neurovascular bundles (NVBs) have become an important part of modern RP. Increasing evidence suggests that the grades of NS are related to the recovery of potency [9–11]. Approaches for the preservation of NVBs can be performed from the prostate base to the apex (antegrade) or from the apex to the base (retrograde). The supposed benefit of the retrograde NS approach over the

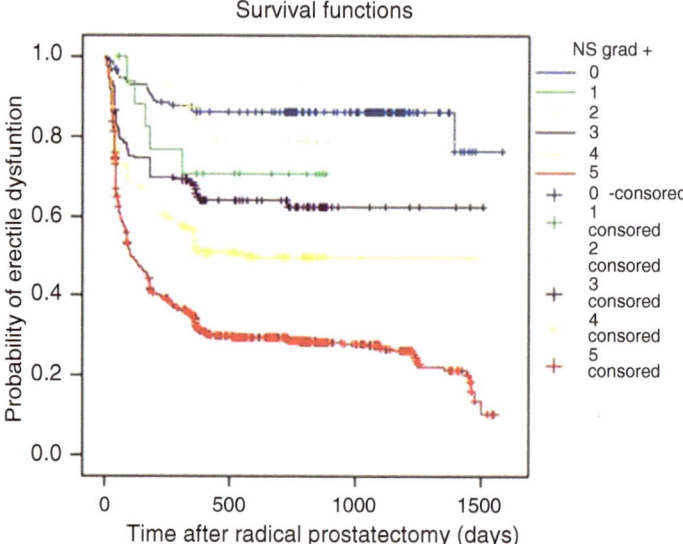

Fig. 6.5 Results of Kaplan–Meier analysis on the probability of erectile dysfunction based on subjective nerve-sparing (NS) grade

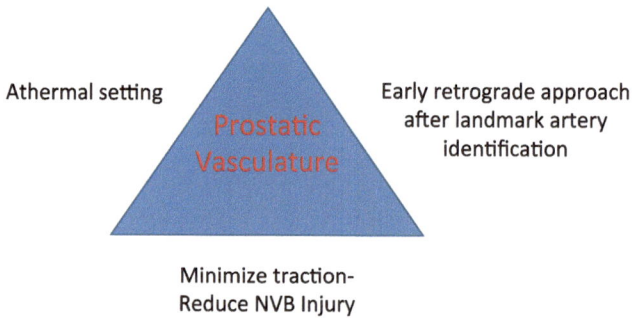

Fig. 6.6 Our approach to neurovascular preservation

antegrade NS approach is the earlier identification and release of the NVB from the prostate before ligating the prostatic pedicle, thus avoiding a misplaced clip on the pedicle. The theoretical benefit of earlier release of the NVB with the pedicle intact is to attenuate neuropraxia [12–14]. Although there is evidence supporting that NS does not affect the positive surgical margin (PSM) rates, the effect of antegrade or retrograde dissection of the NVBs on PSM rates is still unknown [15, 16].

Our group first published comparative results of NS antegrade and retrograde approach demonstrating superiority of the latter one to cause less traction [17]. Based on the data of literature in open retropubic RP and laparoscopic procedure, we suggested athermal retrograde release of the NVBs during RARP.

Antegrade approach: With upward traction of the vasa and seminal vesicles, the prostatic pedicle is identified and athermally controlled close to the base to decrease the risk of severing the NVB. The prostate is then retracted, and the lateral pelvic fascia is exposed. Entering the triangular space between Denonvillier's fascia, the lateral pelvic fascia, and the prostate, the NVB is exposed. Reflecting the lateral pelvic fascia off the prostate, dissection is performed in the interfascial plane, outside the prostatic fascia.

Retrograde approach: After the seminal vesicles have been dissected and the posterior plane is widely developed, the prostate is then rotated and the levator fascia over the prostate is opened sharply to expose the NVB from above. An interfascial plane between the prostate and the NVB is created at the level of the midprostate and is further developed until the previously created posterior plane is reached (Fig. 6.7). The plane is then continued in a retrograde direction toward the base of the prostate to completely detach the NVB from the prostatic pedicle. The plane is then continued toward the apex by detaching the prostate from the NVB.

The computer matched two groups of patients with complete bilateral NS, with no difference between groups, antegrade NS ($n = 172$) and retrograde NS ($n = 172$). Potency rates were evaluated during similar time frames using the SHIM questionnaire. The potency rate was significantly higher in the retrograde NS group than in the antegrade NS group at 3, 6, and 9 months after RARP, without compromising margins status (Fig. 6.8).

Athermal Versus Thermal Dissection of the NVB

The difference between thermal and athermal dissection of the neurovascular bundles (NVB) has been documented extensively [18]. In a 2008 prospective study, Ahlering et al. [19] compared 38 patients receiving cautery nerve sparing with 50 receiving

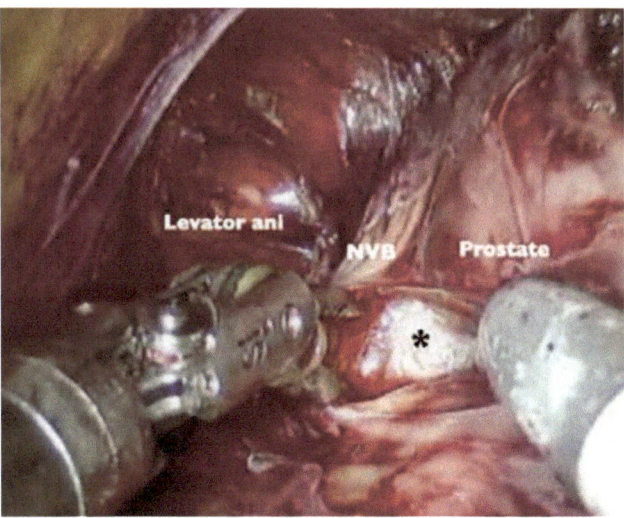

Fig. 6.7 Interfascial plane between the prostate and the NVB

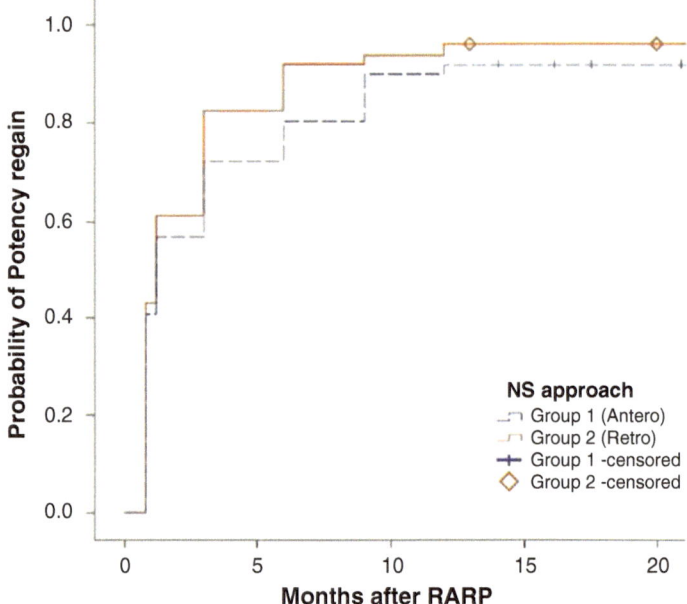

Fig. 6.8 Kaplan–Meier curve for the time to regain potency within a year stratified for each nerve-sparing approach group. The log-rank test indicates the statistically significant difference across each group ($p=0.044$)

cautery-free cavernous nerve preservation. Selecting only patients <65 years of age who were preoperatively potent, the authors reported significant advantages in favor of athermal dissection 24 months after the procedures. In 2010, Samadi et al. [20] compared 590 patients who received an antegrade cautery nerve-sparing procedure using the bipolar device with two other groups of patients who underwent athermal dissection using clips and a "curtain" technique. In this study, including preoperatively potent patients, according to the SHIM questionnaire, with a mean age of 59 years old, the authors showed a statistically significant advantage only in favor of the athermal technique at 3 months follow-up. Any difference disappeared after 6 or 12 months postoperatively.

Considering the data coming from the clinical series reviewed, the mean potency rates at 3, 6, and 12 months were 44 %, 50 %, and 66 % (62–75 %), respectively, in the four series using monopolar or bipolar dissection and 52 %, 78 % (70–86 %), and 81 % (62–90 %), respectively, in the four studies using the athermal dissection. Interestingly, available data with longer follow-up showed a 24-month mean potency rate as high as 82 % (69–94 %) in patients who received cautery nerve sparing.

Nerve-Sparing Technique with Minimal Countertraction

It is well documented that subtle technical variation affects potency preservation during robot-assisted laparoscopic radical prostatectomy (RARP). Most prostatectomy studies focus on achieving the optimal anatomic nerve-sparing dissection plane. However, these sections focus on how the assistant/surgeon neurovascular bundle (NVB) countertraction can impact the sexual function outcomes. Several authors have been able to correlate the effect of countertraction and erectile dysfunction (ED) after RARP. Mulhall et al. [21] identified NVB countertraction as a source of postprostatectomy neurogenic injury. Kaul et al. [22] asserted that endopelvic fascia sparing and delayed DVC ligation reduced NVB traction without mention of assistant or surgeon-specific technique as it relates to NVB tension.

Technique: With an aim of nerve sparing with minimal countertraction (NS-MC), Kowalczyk et al. [13] modified their technique to avoid assistant/surgeon lateral countertraction to dissect the prostate away from the NVB instead of the NVB away from the prostate. Additionally, they decreased robotic scissors excursion with blunt dissection during intrafascial nerve sparing to attenuate tension on the NVB. NS-MC was associated with significantly higher sexual function scores at 5 months after RARP compared to NS countertraction (median: 20 vs 10; $p < 0.001$), been this difference more accentuated for bilateral intrafascial nerve sparing in preoperatively potent men.

New Developments in Minimally Invasive Dissection and Protection NVB During RARP

Human Amniotic Membrane Allograft Nerve Wrap Around the Prostatic Neurovascular Bundle

Clinical use of growth factors and anti-inflammatory substances for prostatic NVB regeneration is novel, and human amnion membrane allograft (dHACM) is a source of implantable neurotrophic factors and cytokines [23, 24]. Since 2014, we implemented a local application of this allograft for preoperatively potent men. The bilateral, retrograde, athermal NS RARP was performed in each patient (Fig. 6.9a), with bladder neck reconstruction, an anterior suspension stitch, and posterior reconstruction (Rocco stitch). There were 58 patients in this series, who were preoperatively continent (American Urological Association Symptom Score <10) and potent (Sexual Health Inventory for Men [SHIM] score >19) and underwent bilateral dHACM placement (AmnioFix; MiMedx Group, Marietta, GA, USA) at a cost of $900 per patient. The dHACM allograft was cut into two longitudinal pieces and placed over each NVB as a nerve wrap. The wrap was placed circumferentially around the NVB after extirpative RARP, postanastomosis (Fig. 6.9b).

This group was computer matched with a similar group of patients who did not receive allograft placement. Postoperative outcomes were analyzed between both groups, including time to return to continence, biochemical recurrence, and potency. Potency at 8 weeks returned in 65.5 % of the patients in the dHACM group and 51.7 % of the patients in the no-dHACM group. The mean time to potency was significantly shorter in the graft group (1.34 months) than in the nongraft group (3.39 months; $p = 0.007$) (Fig. 6.10). SHIM scores were also higher for the dHACM group than for the no-dHACM group (mean score 16.2 vs. 9.1). In conclusion, our short-term results are encouraging for patients undergoing full NS RARP and dHACM placement.

Fig. 6.9 Local application of dHACM allograft after bilateral NS procedure. (**a**) View of bilaterally completely spared both NVBs; (**b**) Left NVB with the dHACM graft on *top*

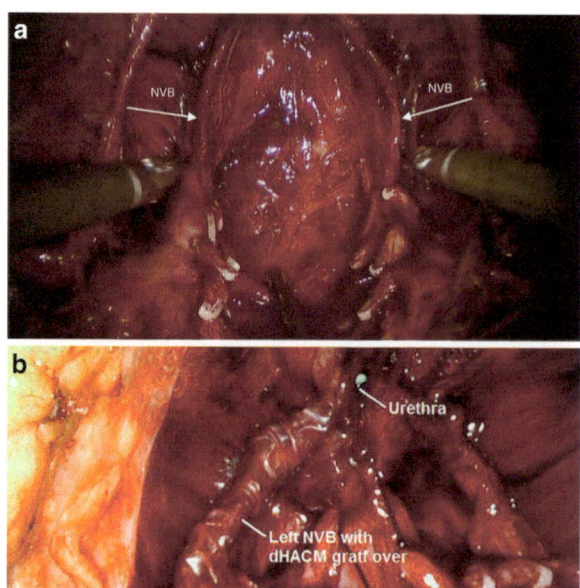

Instant Toggling of Endoscope During RARP

With the introduction of the da Vinci Xi robotic surgical system some of its new applications have been built to try to achieve a more precise sparing procedure. For instance, the laparoscope has a digital end-mounted camera for improved vision. The scope can be placed into any of the robotic arms and has autofocus. The new endoscope is used to see deep inside the body, is far easier to setup and delivers sharp, high-definition 3D images.

We implemented this advanced imaging for clear visualization of the neurovascular bundle to initiate its dissection. The use of maneuver to rotate the 3D camera with 30° lens angles up to 180° can facilitate a more direct view to identify a route of NVB in order to start releasing its dissection from posterior surface (Fig. 6.11a). It is essential to fully dissect the posterior plane up to the apex and laterally to the bundles. Once this is accomplished, early release of NVB can then be performed. At the level of the apex and midportion of the prostate, the avascular plane between the neurovascular bundle and prostatic fascia is developed with caution. Then, the monopolar scissors are used to create the window to separate the prostate from the bundle. By rotating the camera back, it is feasible to maintain an interfacial approach to dissect the anterior and lateral surface of the prostate preserving neurovascular bundle (Fig. 6.11b). Stepwise procedure includes gentle dissection with sweeping motions

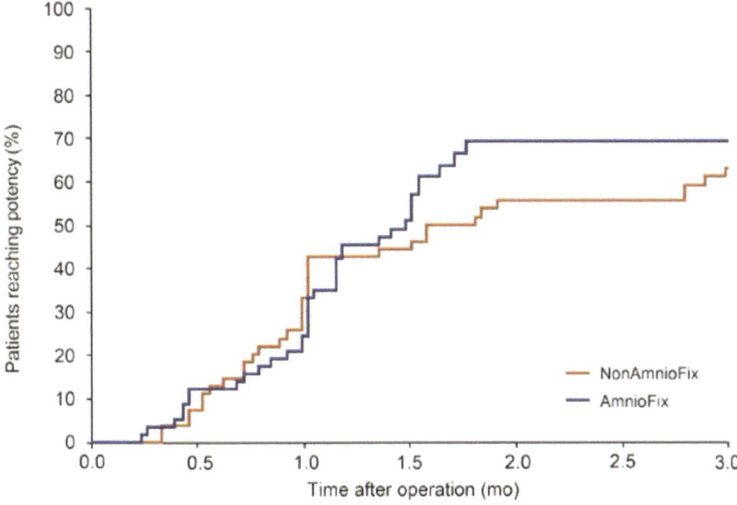

Fig. 6.10 Cumulative index curves showing time to potency. Time to reach potency: AmnioFix group, 1.34 month; non-AmnioFix group, 3.39 months ($p = 0.007$)

of scissors, clear identification of the landmark artery, and gentle dissection with preservation of the neurovascular bundle toward the plane of dissection initiated from the posterior surface before. The retrograde direction facilitates a more anatomical-based plane of dissection toward the prostatic pedicle. The path of the bundle is now delineated and focus can now turn to controlling the prostatic vascular pedicle.

Ultimately, this approach may provide the surgeon with guidance for exact placement of a first hem-o-lock clip to pedicle above the level of the released NVB. This technique allows complete NVB preservation without the use of any thermal energy, significant trauma, or inadvertent damage. Kumar et al. presented results of our first 20 patients using the instant toggling of endoscope during RARP. The mean time for NS was 12.3 min versus 18.1 min in standard procedure ($p < 0.005$). There were no intraoperative/postoperative complications.

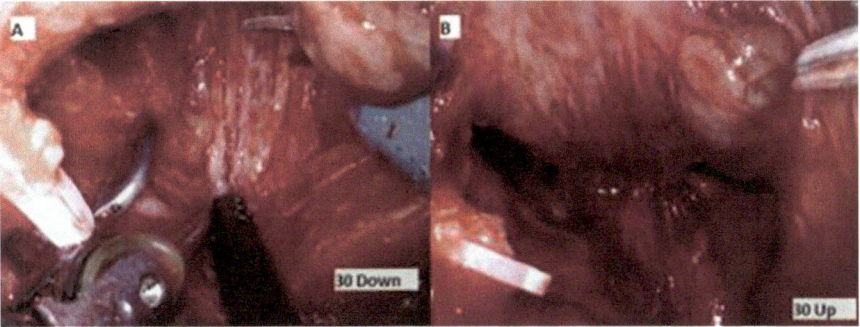

Fig. 6.11 (**A**, **B**) Toggling of camera from 30° down to up. Explanation in the text

The Application of Immunofluorescence as a Novel Optical Imaging Tool to Better Visualize Landmark Artery

Since 2010, a near-infrared fluorescence (NIRF) camera was integrated into the da Vinci Si and the Xi systems, creating a combination of technically and minimally invasive advantages that have been embraced by several experienced surgeons (Fig. 6.12). Commonly used as a contrast agent the Indocyanine Green (ICG) is a vital fluorescent dye characterized by excellent tolerability, few side effects, and low toxicity and allergic reactions. As a result of these characteristics, ICG have been utilized in several fields, in particular to assess microvascular circulation and organ vascularization.

Intraoperatively we injected intravenously 0.75 ml of ICG before pedicle ligation and NVB dissection. The time to target vasculature of prostate was 20–40 s. The technique allowed us to identify the landmark artery in 17/20 (85%) patients (Fig. 6.13). In three patients we were unable to visualize the landmark artery due to large veins overlapping the view.

Penile Rehabilitation After Radical Prostatectomy

Despite the advantages of this new surgical approach, a significant proportion of patients might experience erectile dysfunction, with different degrees of severity.

PDE5 Inhibitors

Since Mulhall et al. [25] first reported the results of penile rehabilitation using sildenafil in 2005, clinical studies have reported that PDE5 inhibitors have protective effects on smooth muscle and endothelial cells, nerve-modulating effects, and inducing effects on corpus cavernosum oxygenation. When sildenafil was administered daily to 76 patients with normal erectile function who had undergone bilateral nerve-sparing

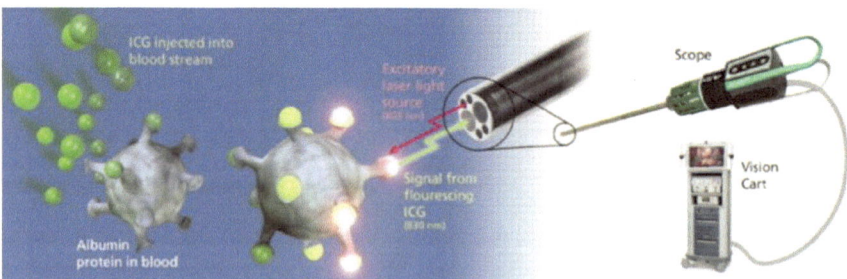

Fig. 6.12 The integration of Immunofluorescence into da Vinci Robot system

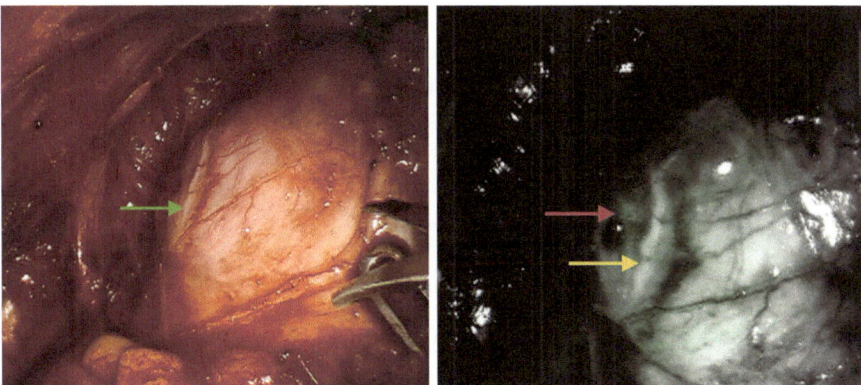

Fig. 6.13 Suspected Landmark Artery (*green arrow*) in the standard robotic view. Firefly view, actual location of the Ladmark Artery (*red arrow*), and the suspected position of the artery on the standard view (*yellow arrow*)

radical prostatectomy 48 weeks earlier, the recovery rate of erectile function was 24 % in the 50 mg dose group, 33 % in the 100 mg dose group, and 5 % in the placebo group. Additionally, when sildenafil was administered to 40 male patients who had undergone bilateral nerve-sparing radical prostatectomies, and a biopsy was conducted before and 6 months after the surgery to compare the effect of sildenafil, no loss of the smooth muscle was seen in the 50 mg dose group, and increased smooth muscle tissue was seen in the 100 mg dose group [26]. Based on these results, we advise our patients to start penile rehabilitative treatment with PDE5 inhibitors soon after surgery.

Intracavernous Injection of Pro-erectile Compound

Intracavernous injection (ICI) of alprostadil represents a valid alternative for patients not responding to PDE5 inhibitors. Claro et al. [27] reported that when intracavernosal injection was conducted on patients who had normal sexual function before curative surgery, but who had postoperative erectile dysfunction, 40 % of the patients showed a good result, and 94.6 % showed erection sufficient to have sexual intercourse. The main disadvantage of ICI relies in the limited compliance to the treatment due to the secondary effects. Penile pain remains the major cause to abandon treatment [28].

Vacuum Constriction Devices

A previous clinical study on the treatment of erectile dysfunction following radical prostatectomy reported that when a vacuum constriction device (VCD) was used for 9 months after the surgery, 80 % of the patients were able to have sex using the device, but only 29 % of the control group members were able to have sex. Another study showed a decrease in penis length by 2 cm in patients who started to use the device 6 months after surgery compared with patients who used the device 1 month after surgery [29]. No large-scale, randomized, controlled study has been reported due to insufficient patient numbers, although we recommend this to our patients in order to prevent penis dystrophy. Chapter 9 discussed penile rehabilitation in more detail.

Published Results

In a multi-institutional prospective analysis of 8000 consecutive cases of robotic-assisted laparoscopic radical prostatectomy according to D'Amico risk criteria [30], the potency rate at 12 months follow-up was 88.4, 79.0, and 60 % in low, intermediate, and high-risk groups, respectively; however, there were no statistically significant differences. Moreover, the overall potency rate ranged from 32.7 to 96.6 %, and similarly, RRP had greater variation (32.7–81.3 %), whereas LRP (64.6 %) and RARP (69–96.6 %) achieved the greater rates. Ninety-four of the 300 patients received a bilateral NVB preservation during RARP, potency was achieved in 87.2 % of the cases.

Our group has also reported our outcomes after RARP. In terms of potency, Patel et al. [31] achieved a 96.6 % of 404 patients, over a follow-up period of 18 months.

Recently, Ficarra et al. [18] summarized results of systematic review and meta-analysis reporting potency rates after RARP when compared with retropubic radical prostatectomy (RRP) and laparoscopic radical prostatectomy (LRP) (Figs. 6.14 and 6.15). Although the initial RARP series showed 12-month potency rates ranging from 70 to 80 %, a lack of comparative studies did not permit any definitive conclusion about the superiority of this technique. Cumulative analyses showed better 12-month potency rates after RARP in comparison with RRP (odds ratio [OR]: 2.84; 95 % confidence interval [CI]: 1.46–5.43; $p = 0.002$) (Fig. 6.14). Only a non-statistically significant trend in favor of RARP was reported after comparison with LRP (OR: 1.89; $p = 0.21$) (Fig. 6.15). This update, for the first time, demonstrated a significant advantage in favor of RARP in comparison with RRP in terms of 12-mo potency rates.

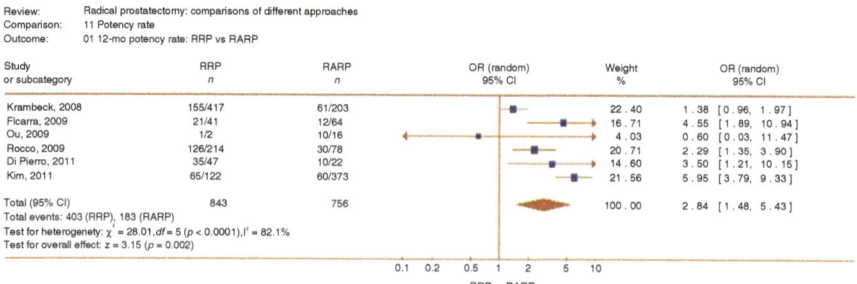

Fig. 6.14 The forest plot of cumulative analysis of 12-month potency rate following RARP versus RRP. *CI* confidence interval, *OD* odds ratio

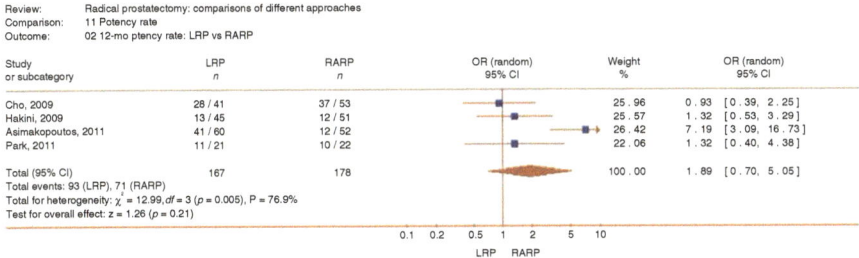

Fig. 6.15 The forest plot of cumulative analysis of 12-month potency rate following RARP versus LRP. *CI* confidence interval, *OD* odds ratio

Conclusion

Nerve-sparing (NS) procedures RARP have demonstrated improved postoperative functional outcomes. We have demonstrated our technique of nerve sparing: athermal, early retrograde release, minimization of tension with identification of landmark artery. We have shown the role of our subjective NS regression model in predicting the recovery time of postoperative erectile function after RARP.

The surgeon's experience and volume are the key determinants in NS RARP. The ICG and NIRF technology during NS RARP has the potential to identify LA accurately and improve the quality of NS. Use of instant toggling of endoscope using Xi da-Vinci robotic surgical system can improve quality of NS in challenging cases of RARP. The dHACM allograft can hasten early return of continence and potency in patients following RARP. However, further multi-institutional long-term randomized controlled trials are required to validate these new findings.

References

1. Walsh PC, Donker PJ. Impotence following radical prostatectomy: insight into etiology and prevention. J Urol. 1982;128:492–7.
2. Tewari A, Peabody JO, Fisher M, et al. An operatives and anatomic study to help in nerve sparing during laparoscopic and robotic radical prostatectomy. Eur Urol. 2003;44:444–54.
3. Flocks RH. The arterial distribution within the prostate gland: its role in transurethral prostatic resection. J Urol. 1937;37:524–48.
4. Clegg EJ. The arterial supply of the human prostate and semnal vesicles. J Anat. 1955;89:209–16.
5. Bilhim T, Pisco JM, Furtado A, et al. Prostatic arterial supply: demonstration by multirow detector angio CT and catheter angiography. Eur Radiol. 2011;21:1119–26.
6. Clegg EJ. The vascular arrangements within the human prostate gland. Br J Urol. 1956;28:428–35.
7. Lepor H, Gregerman M, Crosby R, Mostofi FK, Walsh PC. Precise localization of the autonomic nerves from the pelvic plexus to the corpora cavernosa: a detailed anatomical study of the adult male pelvis. J Urol. 1985;133:207–12.
8. Schatloff O, Chauhan S, Sivaraman A, Kameh D, Palmer K, Patel VR. Anatomic grading of nerve sparing during robot-assisted radical prostatectomy. Eur Urol. 2012;61:796–802.

9. Levinson AW, Pavlovich CP, Ward NT, Link RE, Mettee LZ, Su LM. Association of surgeon subjective characterization of nerve sparing quality with potency following laparoscopic radical prostatectomy. J Urol. 2008;179:1510–4.

10. Dubbelman YD, Dohle GR, Schroder FH. Sexual function before and after radical retropubic prostatectomy: a systematic review of prognostic indicators for a successful outcome. Eur Urol. 2006;50:711–20.

11. van der Poel HG, de Blok W. Role of extent of fascia preservation and erectile function after robot-assisted laparoscopic prostatectomy. Urology. 2009;73:816–21.

12. Coughlin G, Dangle PP, Palmer KJ, Samevedi S, Patel VR. Athermal early retrograde release of the neurovascular bundle during nervesparing robotic-assisted laparoscopic radical prostatectomy. J Robot Surg. 2009;3:13–7.

13. Kowalczyk KJ, Huang AC, Hevelone ND, et al. Stepwise approach for nerve sparing without counterattraction during robot-assisted radical prostatectomy: technique and outcomes. Eur Urol. 2011;60:536–47.

14. Alemozaffar M, Duclos A, Hevelone ND, et al. Technical refinement and learning curve for attenuating neurapraxia during robotic assisted radical prostatectomy to improve sexual function. Eur Urol. 2012;61:1222–8.

15. Ward JF, Zincke H, Bergstralh EJ, Slezak JM, Myers RP, Blute ML. The impact of surgical approach (nerve bundle preservation versus wide local excision) on surgical margins and biochemical recurrence following radical prostatectomy. J Urol. 2004;172:1328–32.

16. Palisaar RJ, Noldus J, Graefen M, Erbersdobler A, Haese A, Huland H. Influence of nervesparing (NS) procedure during radical prostatectomy (RP) on margin status and biochemical failure. Eur Urol. 2005;47:176–84.

17. Ko YH, Coelho RF, Sivaraman A, Schatloff O, Chauhan S, Abdul-Muhsin HM, et al. Retrograde versus antegrade nerve sparing during robotassisted radical prostatectomy: which is better for achieving early functional recovery? Eur Urol. 2013;63:169–77.

18. Ficarra V, Novara G, Ahlering T, et al. Systematic review and meta-analysis of studies reporting potency rates after robot-assisted radical prostatectomy. Eur Urol. 2012;61:418–30.

19. Ahlering TE, Rodriguez E, Skarecky DW. Overcoming obstacles: nerve-sparing issues in radical prostatectomy. J Endourol. 2008;22:745–50.

20. Samadi DB, Muntner P, Nabizada-Pace F, Brajtbord JS, Carlucci J, Lavery HJ. Improvements in robot-assisted prostatectomy: the effect of surgeon experience and technical changes on oncologic and functional outcomes. J Endourol. 2010;24:1105–10.

21. Mulhall JP, Slovick R, Hotaling J, et al. Erectile dysfunction after radical prostatectomy: hemodynamic profiles and their correlation with the recovery of erectile function. J Urol. 2002;167:1371–5.

22. Kaul S, Savera A, Badani K, Fumo M, Bhandari A, Menon M. Functional outcomes and oncological efficacy of Vattikuti Institute prostatectomy with veil of aphrodite nerve sparing: an analysis of 154 consecutive patients. BJU Int. 2006;97:467–72.

23. Liang H, Liang P, Xu Y, Wu J, Liang T, Xu X. DHAM-BMSC matrix promotes axonal regeneration and functional recovery after spinal cord injury in adult rats. J Neurotrauma. 2009;26:1745–57.

24. Quinlan DM, Nelson RJ, Partin AW, Mostwin JL, Walsh PC. The rat as a model for the study of penile erection. J Urol. 1989;141:656–61.

25. Mulhall J, Land S, Parker M, Waters WB, Flanigan RC. The use of an erectogenic pharmacotherapy regimen following radical prostatectomy improves recovery of spontaneous erectile function. J Sex Med. 2005;2:532–40.

26. Schwartz EJ, Wong P, Graydon RJ. Sildenafil preserves intracorporeal smooth muscle after radical retropubic prostatectomy. J Urol. 2004;171:771–4.

27. Claro J de A, de Aboim JE, Maríngolo M, Andrade E, Aguiar W, Nogueira M, et al. Intracavernous injection in the treatment of erectile dysfunction after radical prostatectomy: an observational study. Sao Paulo Med J. 2001;119:135–7.

28. Lakin MM, Montague DK, et al. Intracavernous injection therapy: analysis of results and complications. J Urol. 1990;143:1138–41.
29. Köhler TS, Pedro R, Hendlin K, Utz W, Ugarte R, Reddy P, et al. A pilot study on the early use of the vacuum erection device after radical retropubic prostatectomy. BJU Int. 2007;100:858–62.
30. Ou YC, Yang CK, Wang J, Hung SW, Cheng CL, Tewari AK, et al. The trifecta outcome in 300 consecutive cases of robotic-assisted laparoscopic radical prostatectomy according to D'Amico risk criteria. Eur J Surg Oncol. 2013;39:107–13.
31. Patel VR, Coelho RF, Chauhan S, et al. Continence, potency and oncological outcomes after robotic-assisted radical prostatectomy: early trifecta results of a high-volume surgeon. BJU Int. 2010;106(5):696–702.

Chapter 7
Oncologic Outcomes of Robotic-Assisted Radical Prostatectomy: The "Balancing Act" of Achieving Cancer Control and Minimizing Collateral Damage

P. Sooriakumaran, H.S. Dev, D. Skarecky, Thomas E. Ahlering, and P. Wiklund

Defining Oncologic Outcomes After Radical Prostatectomy

To this day, prostate cancer remains the most common nondermatologic malignancy in Western men, with the vast majority of cases presenting with localized or locally advanced disease [1]. A standard treatment option for this is radical prostatectomy (RP), which was traditionally performed via the open approach, but more recently is typically conducted using robotic assistance (robotic-assisted radical prostatectomy; RARP). As localized/locally advanced prostate cancer has a long natural history, studies examining survival take many years to mature and thus often suffer from low power. Hence, intermediate markers of oncologic outcome have become abundant in the literature, the commonest being biochemical recurrence (BCR). This is defined as a rise in a prostate-specific but not cancer-specific protein called Prostate-Specific Antigen (PSA) released in the blood. While the exact rise that defines BCR is not universally agreed upon, most authorities use a PSA of 0.2 ng/ml or greater [2].

Due to competing causes of mortality in men with BCR post-RP, not all recurrences lead to death, but this measure is regarded as a fairly accurate predictor of

P. Sooriakumaran, BMBS (Hons), MRCS, PhD, FRCSUrol, FEBU (✉)
Nuffield Department of Surgical Sciences, University of Oxford,
Oxford, Oxfordshire OX3 7DQ, UK
e-mail: prasanna.sooriakumaran@nds.ox.ac.uk

H.S. Dev
University of Cambridge, Cambridge, UK

D. Skarecky • T.E. Ahlering
Department of Urology, Irvine Medical Center, University of California, Irvine,
333 The City Drive West, Suite 2100, RT 81, Orange, CA 92868, USA

P. Wiklund, M.D., Ph.D.
Karolinska Institute, Stockholm, Sweden

© Springer International Publishing Switzerland 2016   101
S. Razdan (ed.), *Urinary Continence and Sexual Function After Robotic Radical Prostatectomy*, DOI 10.1007/978-3-319-39448-0_7

prostate cancer-specific mortality and thus used to guide the need for salvage ther-apy [3]. The largest study examined 1997 men postprostatectomy from 1982 to 1997, of which 15% developed BCR. Thirty-five percent of patients with BCR developed metastases after a median of 8 years, and 43% died of prostate cancer, after a median of circa 5 years after metastases [4]. Hence the risk of death from prostate cancer in those with BCR was 15%. A more recent study has quoted a 21% risk of death in men with BCR post-RP, and clearly case-mix is responsible for some of these differences [5]. Regardless, lethal metastatic disease is almost always preceded by a rise in PSA that signifies BCR.

How Positive Surgical Margins Correlate with Oncologic Outcome

A positive surgical margin (PSM) may reflect residual cancer cells at the edge of the surgical resection, and this is a consistent predictor of BCR [6–10]; one study reported a BCR-free survival of 93.8 and 79.9% after adjustment for covariates in those with negative and positive surgical margins, respectively [11]. However, stud-ies directly comparing the effect of a PSM to metastasis-free survival and mortality are much less conclusive. A large registry study of 65,633 patients demonstrated a significant effect of PSM on cancer-specific mortality (HR:1.70 [1.32–2.18]) [10]. Criticism of this work has been directed at the absence of preoperative PSA data, and a recent audit which identified a significant rate of inaccurate coding in the database [12], although a second study has further supported the same conclusions from the SEER database, with PSM affecting mortality after multivariate modeling (HR:1.4 [1.0–1.9]; $p=0.036$) [7]. Nonetheless, some studies which have shown PSM to predict BCR have failed to demonstrate a significant relationship with mor-tality [6, 13, 14]. With such large differences in follow-up, inclusion criteria, and the accurate capture of covariates, it is unsurprising that the literature is conflicting as to whether PSM per se have a direct effect on prostate cancer mortality [15].

What we do know is that the vast majority of studies examining the relationship between PSM and oncologic outcome have done so after open RP. However, RARP has become the market leader in the United States and many other Western nations [16]. Hence, more recent work has sought to compare PSM rates across surgical approaches and to determine the impact on PSM in the RARP population. A meta-analysis based on 400 original articles used propensity score adjustments to demonstrate similar PSM rates for RARP and open RP [17], although a recent retrospective study of over 22,000 RP cases showed superior PSM rates in minimally invasive cases over open RP [18].

Multifocal Margins and Oncologic Outcome

If we accept some of the evidence cited earlier that PSM itself is associated with BCR, we might intuitively expect that multifocal tumors should be at greater risk for more residual tissue to be left behind and BCR to occur more quickly. To this end, a study of 210 men with PSMs revealed a 2.19-fold greater risk of recurrence in those with two or more PSM compared to a unifocal margin [19]. Swanson et al. [20] described an overall crude (unadjusted) recurrence rate across seven recent large case series of 20 % vs. 70 % between unifocal and multifocal disease. However, this result has not been reproduced by larger studies [21, 22], where the additional negative prognostic effect of an additional PSM has not been realized [23]. In a recent review of studies from 2005 to 2011, Fontenot [24] identified three studies where multifocality was found to confer a greater risk of BCR compared to unifocality [25–27], and seven in which no such additive effect was seen [6, 28–30].

The Impact of Margin Length

The impact of margin length would follow similar arguments to the impact of multifocality on BCR outcomes. However, most studies on PSM and BCR in both the open and robotic literature do not report on PSM length and so we are limited to a few reports on which to draw our inferences. Furthermore, studies have generally reduced margin length into a categorical variable, often separating into $<1/\geq1$ mm or $<3/\geq3$ mm. Noting the aforementioned, there have been four recent studies [31–34] which found an increasing PSM length to increase the risk of BCR, while three studies failed to show any significant increase in BCR risk on multivariable analyses [29, 35, 36].

Shikanov and colleagues demonstrated a relationship between PSM length and risk of BCR in 1398 cases of RARP after a median follow-up of 1 year. They were unable to demonstrate an effect of PSM < 1 mm on BCR and postulate that these may represent false positive margins. However, an analysis of 294 RARPs with PSM, which reported margin length as a continuous variable, showed a correlation with BCR across all PSM lengths [31]. A more robust analysis of RARP patients with at least 5 years follow-up established the predictive capability of PSMs ≥3 mm/multifocal margins compared to those <3 mm/unifocal margins (HR:2.84 [1.76–4.59]), and this effect was even more substantial in lower risk cohorts [37].

The Impact of Margin Location

So if margin length is important in predicting oncologic outcome, the next question is whether the site of the PSM matters. If papers dealing with margin length were few and far between, this problem is even greater for the margin location literature, with most studies having insufficient power to pick up any association between margin location and BCR, especially after covariate adjustment or subgroup stratification. The subject is further complicated by inconsistent reporting methods of locations, with the International Society of Urologic Pathologists and the College of American Pathologists proposing different classifications of PSM locations [24]. In general, the following are considered by most investigators to be appropriate descriptors for PSM location [24]:

1. *Apex*: The most distal aspect of the prostate is the most surgically challenging to access especially as we try to maximize preserved urethral length. The prostatic apex passes adjacent to the dorsal venous complex and neurovascular bundles under the pubis [24]. It also presents difficulties during histopathologic analysis because of a sparse 'capsule' which complicates correctly labeling PSMs as organ-confined tumors with an intraprostatic incision (pT2 with PSM); or a margin positive extraprostatic tumor (pT3 with PSM), and risks incorrectly labeling organ-confined tumors (pT2 with negative margin, NSM). Hence, the PSM data at the apex is hugely subjected to the Will Rogers phenomenon in which both pT2 and PT3 PSM rates would be reduced if apical PSMs are reported as pT3 PSM cases due to a lack of a 'capsule' [38]. The apex is considered to be the most common location for PSM across the ORP literature [39]. Although some studies showed a significantly increased risk of BCR with apical PSM after multivariable analysis, others have shown no such relationship [24]; the problem is that prostate cancer that reaches the apex may be indicative of larger tumor volume which may then confound multivariable analyses [40].

2. *Posterolateral and posterior*: Posterolateral margins are the second most common [39] and most often a result of efforts to preserve the neurovascular bundles, as this broadly describes the region where intra-/interfascial dissection occurs for nerve sparing. Three recent reports describe a greater impact on BCR rates with a PSM in this area, while only one failed to demonstrate a significant relationship (of any location including posterolateral) after multivariable regression, likely due to the small sample size [41]. Prostate cancers can also invade posteriorly into Denonvilliers fascia necessitating resection of this posterior fascia. The association between PSM in this region and BCR has also been varied; Fontenot summarized three studies from the last decade which support both conclusions [24].

3. *Base and bladder neck*: The basal prostate refers to the cranial end of the prostate around the bladder neck, although PSM at these sites are often grouped together [34]. PSM here can result from surgical efforts to preserve the bladder neck in an attempt to improve urinary continence recovery. The finding of an isolated PSM at the bladder neck is a reasonably infrequent occurrence (compared to microscopic invasion of the bladder neck, pT3 disease which need not necessarily have an associated PSM). Controversy regarding the impact of PSMs at these sites also exists, particularly for those at the base. Hsu and colleagues reviewed 117 RP patients with positive margins and described a significant impact of bladder neck PSM on BCR (HR:1.29 [1.0–1.67]; $p=0.046$). In contrast, other studies refute the impact of a PSM at the bladder neck on BCR [28, 34, 42].

4. *Anterior*: This is generally considered as a fibromuscular stromal region which is less commonly associated with finding PSMs, with an incidence of 2–15 %. Anterior PSM may be associated with transitional zone tumors and those among the 'anterior horns,' which are at risk of iatrogenic cautery when controlling the surrounding vasculature. This again illustrates the inverse relationship between minimizing collateral damage and PSM rates. The study by Hsu and colleagues also revealed an effect of anterior PSM on BCR (HR:1.17 [1.02–1.33]; $p=0.027$),

possibly as a result of greater iatrogenic intraprostatic incision during vascular control. However, similar to other sites, there remains ambivalence regarding the effect a PSM at this site has on BCR [32, 34, 41, 43, 44].

Differences with the Robotic Approach

One might predict the operative differences of minimally invasive RP may result in a distinct pattern of PSM. A study of 538 patients described the most common PSM site to be in the apical region for ORP (54 %) compared to the posterolateral region (54 %) for laparoscopic RP [45]. Guillonneau [46] reported similar findings with 50 and 30 % at the apex and posterolateral regions, respectively, for their series of 1000 consecutive laparoscopic RP [46]. Similarly, Patel and colleagues reported on 1272 PSMs in 8095 RARP procedures, and in agreement with earlier studies [47] found the apex and posterolateral sites to be the most common PSM locations (36 and 29 %, respectively) [48]. The findings suggest unique technical challenges for intra-operative dissection which may reflect in differing locations of PSM for different surgical approaches.

Sooriakumaran et al. were unable to draw statistically significant conclusions regarding the effect of PSM location on BCR. Initial trends suggest PSM locations in RARP having different prognostic value when compared to ORP, where there is more widely (albeit not completely) accepted importance of posterolateral margins and relative equipoise regarding apical margins [37]. If the fourth arm superomedial traction applied in RARP during nerve sparing is responsible for significantly more intraprostatic incisions, which are considered to have less effect on BCR, then posterolateral margins in RARP should have less oncologic impact than in ORP series.

In order to investigate the impact of PSM parameters (length and location) on BCR after RARP, we conducted a tri-institutional, trans-Atlantic analysis on the topic [49]. Between January 2002 and May 2013 clinicopathologic data on RARP patients was prospectively collected across three participating centers (two US, one Europe). Patients who had received RARP for cT1-3 prostate cancer and did not meet any of the following exclusion criteria were included in this study: not received adjuvant hormonal or radiation therapy; PSA had been recorded for at least 3 years post-RP; and the margin status (presence or absence) of the histopathologic specimen had been recorded. In total, 4001 consecutive patients fulfilled these criteria and were included in this study.

Margin Positive Cases Have Worse Pathologic Stage, Grade, and Preoperative PSA

When comparing a PSM with negative margin cases, chi-squared differences revealed a higher preoperative PSA, smaller prostate volume, and higher stage and grade disease. Thirty-seven percent PSM cases went onto develop BCR compared with just 10 % of negative margin cases.

Posterolateral and Apical Margins Are the Most Common Site of Margin Positivity with RARP

Multifocal, posterolateral, and apical regions contributed to the greatest number of PSMs (27, 27, and 32 %, respectively), and not unexpectedly the largest number of BCR among PSM cases. The highest level of BCR as a proportion was found at the base, with over half of all margins (19 of 35) producing BCR.

A Positive Margin Adversely Affects Outcome

On univariate binary logistic regression analysis, margin positivity at the base demonstrated a 10.2× greater risk of BCR, compared to the 3–4× odds ratio for the other locations. The effect however was lost on multivariate analysis, and similarly institution, BMI and age become nonsignificant when covariates are included. However, the odds for BCR with a PSM vs. NSM remained prominent: OR:3.1 c.f. OR:4.2 for stage $\geq$pT3b c.f. OR:1.3 for preoperative PSA.

A Positive Margin at Any Location Favors BCR

All margin locations had a significantly greater chance than negative margins of resulting in BCR, with a trend in odds ratios favoring anterior and apical margins as predictors of BCR compared to margins at the base or posterolaterally (odds ratios: 3.36, 3. 27, 3.01, and 2.97, respectively).

PSM and Margin Length $\geq$3 mm Has a Greater Effect on BCR in Lower Risk Cohorts

Multivariate cox regression identified an instantaneous hazard ratio of 1.85 for PSM vs. NSM leading to BCR. Stratification by pathologic stage ($\leq$pT2 vs. $\geq$pT3) and Gleason grade ($\leq$3+4 vs. $\geq$4+3) revealed a substantially greater impact of a PSM in lower risk cohorts: 3.06 vs. 1.58 and 2.35 vs. 1.67, respectively (all $p < 0.001$). This holds true for margin length, with PSM$\geq$3 mm having almost double the effect of $\leq$3 mm on BCR in lower risk cohorts compared to all risk cohorts taken together.

Apical Margins Are More Hazardous Than Posterolateral Margins

Propensity adjusted cox regression analysis revealed significant hazard ratios across all margin locations. Although the magnitude of the instantaneous risk of BCR differs between statistical models, the trend for apical locations to show *greater* effects across these multivariable models was noteworthy, particularly when compared to posterolateral margins: 3.54 vs. 2.837 (on propensity adjusted Cox regression); 2.334

vs. 1.685 (on multivariate Cox regression); 3.272 vs. 2.966 (on binary logistic model). Hence apical margins appeared to have a greater hazard of BCR than posterolateral margins, after statistical analysis based on a common reference (NSM).

Discussion

Our study found that PSM are associated with a greater risk of BCR after RARP compared to negative margins. This concurs with growing evidence across open series, and recent minimally invasive series [28, 48]. It is perhaps not surprising that some of this effect is by association, and we see PSM associated with other risk factors for BCR such as tumor grade and stage.

We demonstrated the greater impact PSM carries on lower risk (pT2 or Gleason $\leq 3+4$ or both) prostate cancers after subgroup analysis. This probably reflects a relative balance with other more influential factors. Gleason grade and tumor stage probably have the largest impact on risk of BCR [48, 50, 51], although PSM remains the most important 'surgically controllable' predictor of BCR. Indeed, the presence of a PSM is itself dependent on some of these factors, most notably pathologic stage; incidence of PSM has been reported as 9 % for pT2, 37 % for pT3, and 50 % for pT4 [52]. So this is the crux of the issue: with high grade and stage tumors, the biology of the disease drives the risk of BCR with margin status having little independent predictive value over and beyond the biologic variables. However, with low risk tumors in which biology is unlikely to lead to BCR, the relative increased risk of relapse with a PSM compared with a negative margin is much greater. A report on nearly 1000 cases from the Karolinska University Hospital (Stockholm, Sweden) on men with at least 5 years of follow-up post-RARP confirms these findings [53].

The counterpoint of this argument is that the absolute risk of BCR is much higher for high grade and stage tumors than for low ones, and thus any increased risk of relapse may be considered to be more important for the former cases. From the oncologic perspective, it might thus be more imperative for the surgeon to attempt to get a negative margin at the cost of increasing collateral damage in these high-risk cases and be less concerned with getting negative margins in cases of low Gleason grade or stage. Here, the surgeon might choose to accept higher PSM for minimizing collateral damage and thus optimizing the functional outcomes of urinary continence recovery and erectile function. This is the balancing act that becomes the surgeon's edict. With nerve sparing during RARP most likely to lead to PSM in the posterolateral region, and our work described herein that suggests this has minimal impact on BCR, surgeons should not shy away from aggressive nerve sparing for low-risk RARP cases. This is even more important given recent data that the more aggressive the nerve sparing, the better the continence as well as erectile outcomes are [54].

Hazard ratios from our statistical modeling appear to suggest a weaker impact of posterolateral margins on BCR compared to other sites, and this is particularly surprising when compared to evidence from open RP, where the impact of posterolateral PSM on BCR is well established [39]. Indeed, Vickers and colleagues have described posterolateral PSM in pT2 disease as an adverse factor on outcome, and related to inadequate surgical technique [55].

The lack of tactile feedback which results from operating with a robotic platform has long been cited as a potential reason for greater iatrogenic PSM. However, many have reported the use of visual cues to offset any loss in tactile feedback and comparing crude PSM rates between studies seems to suggest fewer may be caused by robotic compared to open operations [56, 57]. That said, one hypothesis regarding posterolateral margins is the fourth arm robotic traction places on the prostatic 'capsule' and surrounding structures, particularly during craniomedial elevation of the vasa/seminal vesicles during posterolateral dissection. The sustained tension resulting from hitching up the prostate, particularly during prolonged periods when performing nerve sparing, is likely to facilitate easier dissection but perhaps also causes iatrogenic intraprostatic incisions. Secin and colleagues found a counterintuitive relationship between PSM and extrafascial nerve-sparing procedure, possibly resulting from a technical error forcing false planes and producing capsular flaps [15], although we did not have the 'nerve-sparing' status as a variable for our analysis.

In a study of 2442 patients, Eastham and colleagues describe a significant impact of posterolateral margin status on BCR (HR: 2.8 [1.76-4.44]), but failed to demonstrate an effect of apical margins (HR0.94 [0.59–1.51]). Eastham comments on a higher risk of BCR in open RP series with posterolateral margins, as the area least likely to receive iatrogenic trauma as well as its proximity to nerves which permits perineural invasion [3]. They instead suggest the apex is under greater traction with false positive margins, less supporting tissue at the apex providing less vascular support for metastatic spread [3]. While this cannot be discounted, this likely reflects the open surgical technique. Clearly, targeted traction of the robotic instruments around the prostate to facilitate nerve sparing can still cause iatrogenic damage while sparing the neurovasculature from direct injury.

Pettus and Pfitzenmaier have described a significant impact of apical PSM on BCR [9, 23], although Pettus's analysis fails on multivariate analysis; several other earlier studies including one of 172 patients over 3½ years follow-up also failed to demonstrate an association between apical PSMs and clinical progression [58, 59].

The findings of our study suggest apical margins are more hazardous than posterolateral ones in RARP and support a trend seen in one recent study [37]. While the apex has been shown to impact BCR in some studies from ORP series, this effect is often less than a PSM elsewhere. While our study did not directly compare ORP and RARP cases, the dominance of apical margin positivity associated with BCR has not been seen before in RARP series, and technical differences between the two surgical approaches must be considered at least partially responsible. Intraoperative differences in terms of approach, traction, and risk of iatrogenic capsular incisions are likely to be responsible for these differences.

Two of the three institutions involved in our multi-institutional study have made specific efforts toward altering their control of the dorsal venous complex prior to attempting apical dissection. Theories as to why the order of these two operative steps may affect apical PSM rates include the possible effect of bunching up tissue around the apex and distorting apical anatomy. Alternative methods (supported by the third institution of our study) advocate division of these vessels prior to apical dissection which would encourage more inferior incisions in an effort to avoid the dorsal veins and blood loss, which might inadvertently lead to an intraprostatic incision [37, 60, 61]. The apex is a technically challenging region to operate in, particularly with variations in shape. Technical modifications however continue to improve PSM rates, particularly at the apex, with variations in the RARP technique, e.g., retroapical approach [56], allowing better circumferential visualization of the apex and membranous urethra, leading to a total decrease as well as proportionally fewer apical margins as a percentage of total PSM burden. Because of these efforts it should therefore follow that the PSMs that will remain at the apex are biologically rather than surgically attributable PSM (i.e., fewer false positives) which would thus carry a worse prognosis.

Ergo, there are fewer apical margins evident with this technique, due to less false negative iatrogenic damage to the apex. Although there were 27.5 % margins classified as apical in our study, we do not have an open RP arm to compare with, and comparisons in the context of such a wide range of values in the literature are unhelpful. However, it remains possible that this reflects an increasingly smaller percentage of false positive margins as a result of improved technical dissection using the robotic platform.

A failure to identify capsular incisions from pT3 PSM at the apex would falsely upstage the disease (Will Rogers phenomenon) and also lead to lower than expected impact of the apical margin location when taking into account other variables in multivariable models. If carcinoma extends to the inked margin adjacent to benign prostatic glands, and in the absence of adipocytes, this can be used to differentiate PSM at the apex with associated extraprostatic extension (EPE). However, there is no consensus as to a reliable method to make this distinction and many authors do not routinely diagnose EPE at the apex for this reason [62].

Understaging can also result from a phenomenon of fibrotic desmoplastic reaction following extraprostatic extension, and can confuse any assessment of margin status, and this may lead to ascribing more importance to apical margins; although suggestions have been made that this occurs in the posterolateral region, which would further strengthen our findings of a difference between these locations [39].

We generally found higher hazard ratios associated with anterior and apical margins compared to posterolateral and basal ones, although the numbers involved at these sites were smaller. The anterior prostate is predominantly fibromuscular stroma and a PSM here may reflect inherent aggressiveness of any tumor able to migrate into it (rather than necessarily reflecting a site of origin which is innately aggressive—see earlier). It is also possible the close proximity to vasculature provides a more favorable location for distant spread.

Suggestions for future approaches to prevent PSM, beyond technical modifications, have included routine intraoperative frozen sections to permit secondary resection intraoperatively; 25 % of cases are found to detect residual cancer on attempts at removing further tissue, implying a PSM may not always reflect residual cancer in the prostatic bed [63]. Follow-up data is lacking regarding the effect on outcomes such as BCR rates in those treated using this method.

Conclusions

PSMs remain a critical finding to identify and better understand, given its profound patient implications in terms of prognosis and further treatment. All PSMs resulting from RARP are not equivalent; longer margins suggest a higher risk of recurrence and the influence is especially prominent in lower risk patients. The apex is a significant contributor to BCR and appears to have the strongest impact of all the margin locations in RARP patients. In contrast, the posterolateral region appears to carry a smaller effect on BCR, probably reflecting greater iatrogenic injury to the prostate in this region. Hence, RARP surgeons might choose to accept the increased risk of posterolateral margins during nerve sparing in lower grade and stage prostate cancer patients, but rather make a wider dissection in the higher risk cases sacrificing functional outcomes for lower PSM in these men.

References

1. Orr DP, Fineberg NS, Gray DL. Glycemic control and transfer of health care among adolescents with insulin dependent diabetes mellitus. J Adolesc Health. 1996;18(1):44–7.
2. Heidenreich A, Bastian PJ, Bellmunt J, Bolla M, Joniau S, van der Kwast T, et al. EAU guidelines on prostate cancer. Part II: treatment of advanced, relapsing, and castration-resistant prostate cancer. Eur Urol. 2014;65(2):467–79.
3. Eastham JA, Kuroiwa K, Ohori M, Serio AM, Gorbonos A, Maru N, et al. Prognostic significance of location of positive margins in radical prostatectomy specimens. Urology. 2007;70(5):965–9.
4. Freedland SJ, Humphreys EB, Mangold LA, Eisenberger M, Dorey FJ, Walsh PC, et al. Risk of prostate cancer-specific mortality following biochemical recurrence after radical prostatectomy. JAMA. 2005;294(4):433–9.
5. Antonarakis ES, Chen Y, Elsamanoudi SI, Brassell SA, Da Rocha MV, Eisenberger MA, et al. Long-term overall survival and metastasis-free survival for men with prostate-specific antigen-recurrent prostate cancer after prostatectomy: analysis of the Center for Prostate Disease Research National Database. BJU Int. 2011;108(3):378–85.
6. Boorjian SA, Karnes RJ, Crispen PL, Carlson RE, Rangel LJ, Bergstralh EJ, et al. The impact of positive surgical margins on mortality following radical prostatectomy during the prostate specific antigen era. J Urol. 2010;183(3):1003–9.
7. Chalfin HJ, Dinizo M, Trock BJ, Feng Z, Partin AW, Walsh PC, et al. Impact of surgical margin status on prostate-cancer-specific mortality. BJU Int. 2012;110(11):1684–9.
8. Mauermann J, Fradet V, Lacombe L, Dujardin T, Tiguert R, Tetu B, et al. The impact of solitary and multiple positive surgical margins on hard clinical end points in 1712 adjuvant treatment-naive pT2-4 N0 radical prostatectomy patients. Eur Urol. 2013;64(1):19–25.
9. Pfitzenmaier J, Pahernik S, Tremmel T, Haferkamp A, Buse S, Hohenfellner M. Positive surgical margins after radical prostatectomy: do they have an impact on biochemical or clinical progression? BJU Int. 2008;102(10):1413–8.
10. Wright JL, Dalkin BL, True LD, Ellis WJ, Stanford JL, Lange PH, et al. Positive surgical margins at radical prostatectomy predict prostate cancer specific mortality. J Urol. 2010;183(6):2213–8.
11. Alkhateeb S, Alibhai S, Fleshner N, Finelli A, Jewett M, Zlotta A, et al. Impact of positive surgical margins after radical prostatectomy differs by disease risk group. J Urol. 2010;183(1):145–50.
12. Shah SK, Fleet TM, Williams V, Smith AY, Skipper B, Wiggins C. SEER coding standards result in underestimation of positive surgical margin incidence at radical prostatectomy: results of a systematic audit. J Urol. 2011;186(3):855–9.

13. Stephenson AJ, Eggener SE, Hernandez AV, Klein EA, Kattan MW, Wood Jr DP, et al. Do margins matter? The influence of positive surgical margins on prostate cancer-specific mortality. Eur Urol. 2014;65(4):675–80.

14. Eggener SE, Scardino PT, Walsh PC, Han M, Partin AW, Trock BJ, et al. Predicting 15-year prostate cancer specific mortality after radical prostatectomy. J Urol. 2011;185(3):869–75.

15. Yossepowitch O, Briganti A, Eastham JA, Epstein J, Graefen M, Montironi R, et al. Positive surgical margins after radical prostatectomy: a systematic review and contemporary update. Eur Urol. 2014;65(2):303–13.

16. Trinh QD, Sammon J, Sun M, Ravi P, Ghani KR, Bianchi M, et al. Perioperative outcomes of robot-assisted radical prostatectomy compared with open radical prostatectomy: results from the nationwide inpatient sample. Eur Urol. 2012;61(4):679–85.

17. Tewari A, Sooriakumaran P, Bloch DA, Seshadri-Kreaden U, Hebert AE, Wiklund P. Positive surgical margin and perioperative complication rates of primary surgical treatments for prostate cancer: a systematic review and meta-analysis comparing retropubic, laparoscopic, and robotic prostatectomy. Eur Urol. 2012;62(1):1–15.

18. Sooriakumaran P, John M, Wiklund P, Lee D, Nilsson A, Tewari AK. Learning curve for robotic assisted laparoscopic prostatectomy: a multi-institutional study of 3794 patients. Minerva Urol Nefrol. 2011;63(3):191–8.

19. Sofer M, Hamilton-Nelson KL, Civantos F, Soloway MS. Positive surgical margins after radical retropubic prostatectomy: the influence of site and number on progression. J Urol. 2002;167(6):2453–6.

20. Swanson GP, Lerner SP. Positive margins after radical prostatectomy: implications for failure and role of adjuvant treatment. Urol Oncol. 2013;31(5):531–41.

21. Kausik SJ, Blute ML, Sebo TJ, Leibovich BC, Bergstralh EJ, Slezak J, et al. Prognostic significance of positive surgical margins in patients with extraprostatic carcinoma after radical prostatectomy. Cancer. 2002;95(6):1215–9.

22. Grossfeld GD, Chang JJ, Broering JM, Miller DP, Yu J, Flanders SC, et al. Impact of positive surgical margins on prostate cancer recurrence and the use of secondary cancer treatment: data from the CaPSURE database. J Urol. 2000;163(4):1171–7. quiz 295.

23. Pettus JA, Weight CJ, Thompson CJ, Middleton RG, Stephenson RA. Biochemical failure in men following radical retropubic prostatectomy: impact of surgical margin status and location. J Urol. 2004;172(1):129–32.

24. Fontenot PA, Mansour AM. Reporting positive surgical margins after radical prostatectomy: time for standardization. BJU Int. 2013;111(8):E290–9.

25. Stephenson AJ, Wood DP, Kattan MW, Klein EA, Scardino PT, Eastham JA, et al. Location, extent and number of positive surgical margins do not improve accuracy of predicting prostate cancer recurrence after radical prostatectomy. J Urol. 2009;182(4):1357–63.

26. Resnick MJ, Canter DJ, Guzzo TJ, Magerfleisch L, Tomaszewski JE, Brucker BM, et al. Defining pathological variables to predict biochemical failure in patients with positive surgical margins at radical prostatectomy: implications for adjuvant radiotherapy. BJU Int. 2010;105(10):1377–80.

27. Kordan Y, Salem S, Chang SS, Clark PE, Cookson MS, Davis R, et al. Impact of positive apical surgical margins on likelihood of biochemical recurrence after radical prostatectomy. J Urol. 2009;182(6):2695–701.

28. Shikanov S, Song J, Royce C, Al-Ahmadie H, Zorn K, Steinberg G, et al. Length of positive surgical margin after radical prostatectomy as a predictor of biochemical recurrence. J Urol. 2009;182(1):139–44.

29. May M, Brookman-May S, Weissbach L, Herbst H, Gilfrich C, Papadopoulos T, et al. Solitary and small (</=3 mm) apical positive surgical margins are related to biochemical recurrence after radical prostatectomy. Int J Urol. 2011;18(4):282–9.

30. Budaus L, Isbarn H, Eichelberg C, Lughezzani G, Sun M, Perrotte P, et al. Biochemical recurrence after radical prostatectomy: multiplicative interaction between surgical margin status and pathological stage. J Urol. 2010;184(4):1341–6.

31. Cao D, Humphrey PA, Gao F, Tao Y, Kibel AS. Ability of linear length of positive margin in radical prostatectomy specimens to predict biochemical recurrence. Urology. 2011;77(6):1409–14.

32. Hsu M, Chang SL, Ferrari M, Nolley R, Presti Jr JC, Brooks JD. Length of site-specific positive surgical margins as a risk factor for biochemical recurrence following radical prostatectomy. Int J Urol. 2011;18(4):272–9.
33. Brimo F, Partin AW, Epstein JI. Tumor grade at margins of resection in radical prostatectomy specimens is an independent predictor of prognosis. Urology. 2010;76(5):1206–9.
34. Savdie R, Horvath LG, Benito RP, Rasiah KK, Haynes AM, Chatfield M, et al. High Gleason grade carcinoma at a positive surgical margin predicts biochemical failure after radical prostatectomy and may guide adjuvant radiotherapy. BJU Int. 2012;109(12):1794–800.
35. Psutka SP, Feldman AS, Rodin D, Olumi AF, Wu CL, McDougal WS. Men with organ-confined prostate cancer and positive surgical margins develop biochemical failure at a similar rate to men with extracapsular extension. Urology. 2011;78(1):121–5.
36. Marks RA, Koch MO, Lopez-Beltran A, Montironi R, Juliar BE, Cheng L. The relationship between the extent of surgical margin positivity and prostate specific antigen recurrence in radical prostatectomy specimens. Hum Pathol. 2007;38(8):1207–11.
37. Sooriakumaran P, Ploumidis A, Nyberg T, Olsson M, Akre O, Haendler L, et al. The impact of length and location of positive margins in predicting biochemical recurrence after robotic-assisted radical prostatectomy with a minimum follow-up time of five years. BJU Int. 2013.
38. Gofrit ON, Zorn KC, Steinberg GD, Zagaja GP, Shalhav AL. The Will Rogers phenomenon in urological oncology. J Urol. 2008;179(1):28–33.
39. Meeks JJ, Eastham JA. Radical prostatectomy: positive surgical margins matter. Urol Oncol. 2013;31(7):974–9.
40. Ohori M, Abbas F, Wheeler TM, Kattan MW, Scardino PT, Lerner SP. Pathological features and prognostic significance of prostate cancer in the apical section determined by whole mount histology. J Urol. 1999;161(2):500–4.
41. Saether T, Sorlien LT, Viset T, Lydersen S, Angelsen A. Are positive surgical margins in radical prostatectomy specimens an independent prognostic marker? Scand J Urol Nephrol. 2008;42(6):514–21.
42. Anastasiou I, Tyritzis SI, Adamakis I, Mitropoulos D, Stravodimos KG, Katafigiotis I, et al. Prognostic factors identifying biochemical recurrence in patients with positive margins after radical prostatectomy. Int Urol Nephrol. 2011;43(3):715–20.
43. Godoy G, Tareen BU, Lepor H. Site of positive surgical margins influences biochemical recurrence after radical prostatectomy. BJU Int. 2009;104(11):1610–4.
44. Bastide C, Savage C, Cronin A, Zelefsky MJ, Eastham JA, Touijer K, et al. Location and number of positive surgical margins as prognostic factors of biochemical recurrence after salvage radiation therapy after radical prostatectomy. BJU Int. 2010;106(10):1454–7.
45. Salomon L, Anastasiadis AG, Levrel O, Katz R, Saint F, de la Taille A, et al. Location of positive surgical margins after retropubic, perineal, and laparoscopic radical prostatectomy for organ-confined prostate cancer. Urology. 2003;61(2):386–90.
46. Guillonneau B, el-Fettouh H, Baumert H, Cathelineau X, Doublet JD, Fromont G, et al. Laparoscopic radical prostatectomy: oncological evaluation after 1,000 cases a Montsouris Institute. J Urol. 2003;169(4):1261–6.
47. Smith Jr JA, Chan RC, Chang SS, Herrell SD, Clark PE, Baumgartner R, et al. A comparison of the incidence and location of positive surgical margins in robotic assisted laparoscopic radical prostatectomy and open retropubic radical prostatectomy. J Urol. 2007;178(6):2385–9. discussion 9-90.
48. Patel VR, Coelho RF, Rocco B, Orvieto M, Sivaraman A, Palmer KJ, et al. Positive surgical margins after robotic assisted radical prostatectomy: a multi-institutional study. J Urol. 2011;186(2):511–6.
49. Dev HS, Wiklund P, Patel V, Parashar D, Palmer K, Nyberg T, et al. Surgical margin length and location affect recurrence rates after robotic prostatectomy. Urol Oncol. 2015;33(3):109.e7–13.
50. Kasraeian A, Barret E, Chan J, Sanchez-Salas R, Validire P, Cathelineau X, et al. Comparison of the rate, location and size of positive surgical margins after laparoscopic and robot-assisted laparoscopic radical prostatectomy. BJU Int. 2011;108(7):1174–8.

51. Fleshner NE, Evans A, Chadwick K, Lawrentschuk N, Zlotta A. Clinical significance of the positive surgical margin based upon location, grade, and stage. Urol Oncol. 2010;28(2):197–204.
52. Novara G, Ficarra V, Mocellin S, Ahlering TE, Carroll PR, Graefen M, et al. Systematic review and meta-analysis of studies reporting oncologic outcome after robot-assisted radical prostatectomy. Eur Urol. 2012;62(3):382–404.
53. Sooriakumaran P, Haendler L, Nyberg T, Gronberg H, Nilsson A, Carlsson S, et al. Biochemical recurrence after robot-assisted radical prostatectomy in a European single-centre cohort with a minimum follow-up time of 5 years. Eur Urol. 2012;62(5):768–74.
54. Srivastava A, Chopra S, Pham A, Sooriakumaran P, Durand M, Chughtai B, et al. Effect of a risk-stratified grade of nerve-sparing technique on early return of continence after robot-assisted laparoscopic radical prostatectomy. Eur Urol. 2013;63(3):438–44.
55. Vickers AJ, Bianco FJ, Gonen M, Cronin AM, Eastham JA, Schrag D, et al. Effects of pathologic stage on the learning curve for radical prostatectomy: evidence that recurrence in organ-confined cancer is largely related to inadequate surgical technique. Eur Urol. 2008;53(5):960–6.
56. Tewari AK, Srivastava A, Mudaliar K, Tan GY, Grover S, El Douaihy Y, et al. Anatomical retro-apical technique of synchronous (posterior and anterior) urethral transection: a novel approach for ameliorating apical margin positivity during robotic radical prostatectomy. BJU Int. 2010;106(9):1364–73.
57. Sooriakumaran P, Srivastava A, Shariat SF, Stricker PD, Ahlering T, Eden CG, et al. A multinational, multi-institutional study comparing positive surgical margin rates among 22393 open, laparoscopic, and robot-assisted radical prostatectomy patients. Eur Urol. 2013.
58. van den Ouden D, Bentvelsen FM, Boeve ER, Schroder FH. Positive margins after radical prostatectomy: correlation with local recurrence and distant progression. Br J Urol. 1993;72(4):489–94.
59. Fesseha T, Sakr W, Grignon D, Banerjee M, Wood Jr DP, Pontes JE. Prognostic implications of a positive apical margin in radical prostatectomy specimens. J Urol. 1997;158(6):2176–9.
60. Patel VR, Thaly R, Shah K. Robotic radical prostatectomy: outcomes of 500 cases. BJU Int. 2007;99(5):1109–12.
61. Ahlering TE, Woo D, Eichel L, Lee DI, Edwards R, Skarecky DW. Robot-assisted versus open radical prostatectomy: a comparison of one surgeon's outcomes. Urology. 2004;63(5):819–22.
62. Tan PH, Cheng L, Srigley JR, Griffiths D, Humphrey PA, van der Kwast TH, et al. International Society of Urological Pathology (ISUP) consensus conference on handling and staging of radical prostatectomy specimens. Working group 5: surgical margins. Mod Pathol. 2011;24(1):48–57.
63. von Bodman C, Brock M, Roghmann F, Byers A, Loppenberg B, Braun K, et al. Intraoperative frozen section of the prostate decreases positive margin rate while ensuring nerve sparing procedure during radical prostatectomy. J Urol. 2013;190(2):515–20.

Chapter 8
Adjunctive Measures and New Therapies to Optimize Early Return of Urinary Continence

Rose Khavari and Brian J. Miles

Introduction

In the era of robotically assisted laparoscopic prostatectomy despite the powerful visualization, refined surgical techniques, minimal blood loss, and multiple nerve-sparing and reconstructive bladder neck techniques, urinary incontinence still creates a significant burden on patients and their treating physicians. Chapter 5 focuses on the preoperative, intraoperative, and postoperative technical and surgical skills and modifications that may improve urinary continence in the early and late post-prostatectomy period. In this chapter, we review the literature on nonsurgical interventions that may improve urinary continence in the short near term. Return of urinary continence as reported in the literature varies considerably, depending on surgeon expertise, definition, surgical volume (of both the surgeon and the hospital/medical center), and whether or not the outcome is patient or surgeon reported. Furthermore, the incidence of urinary incontinence experienced by men prior to prostatectomy is generally not recorded and not well known. For instance, Johnson and Ouslander reported 15–30 % of men over age 65 had urinary incontinence to some degree before undergoing radical prostatectomy [1].

Predictors of Urinary Continence Following Prostatectomy

For the past 50 years, urologists have been investigating risk factors that could predict urinary continence outcomes following radical prostatectomy. Knowledge of these risk factors may help surgeons counsel patients more appropriately preoperatively and

R. Khavari, M.D. • B.J. Miles, M.D. (✉)
Urology, Weill Cornell Medical College, 6565 Fannin Suite 200, Houston, TX 77030, USA
e-mail: bjmiles@houstonmethodist.org

© Springer International Publishing Switzerland 2016   115
S. Razdan (ed.), *Urinary Continence and Sexual Function After Robotic Radical Prostatectomy*, DOI 10.1007/978-3-319-39448-0_8

consider earlier and more aggressive interventions. Kumar et al. retrospectively analyzed their prospective collected data on 3362 patients with 1-year follow-up who have undergone robotic-assisted radical prostatectomy stratifying them to six groups: Group I, age more than 70; Group II, BMI 35 and over; Group III, prior bladder neck procedures; Group IV, prostate weight equal to or more than 80 g; Group V, salvage prostatectomy; and finally Group VI, with none of the above risk factors. Interestingly, the authors demonstrated that selected risk factors such as age, prostate weight, BMI, and prior bladder neck procedures only adversely affected the time to return to continence not the continence rate. Nevertheless, salvage prostatectomy patients showed to have a significantly lower continence rates in addition to delayed in mean time to return to continence [2].

In another smaller study with a shorter follow-up of 1 month from Canada, 327 patients who had undergone robotic-assisted radical prostatectomy were prospectively evaluated for predictors of early continence. The authors investigated prostate-specific antigen, prostate weight, International Prostate Symptom Score (IPSS), Sexual Health Inventory for Men (SHIM) score, and type of nerve sparing performed as potential contributing risk factors in early continence. Advanced age and IPSS scores were independent predictors of early continence following robotic radical prostatectomy in this limited patient population suggesting that significant lower urinary tract symptoms can negatively affect the path to continence postsurgery [3].

Other investigators have created a predictive model of urinary continence recovery after radical prostatectomy that incorporates magnetic resonance imaging data (membranous urethral length) and clinical contributors (age, BMI, and American Society of Anesthesiologists score) [4]. In a large group studied by Holm et al., 844 patients were prospectively evaluated for patients' ratings and risk factors for urinary continence following 12 months follow-up. The authors reported a considerable variation in reporting continence depending on the definition applied for urinary incontinence. They also reported that age more than 65, not working, sexual dysfunction, and preoperative urinary incontinence were strong predictors for postprostatectomy incontinence [5].

These risk stratifications not only can be used to counsel patients preoperatively appropriately for their continence expectations following prostatectomy but also encourage early intervention in the high-risk group.

Pathophysiology of Lower Urinary Tract Symptoms

In order to understand what adjunctive measures may influence the path to continence, we need to understand how the pelvic floor, urethral anatomy, and function change following radical prostatectomy. Chapter 1 reviews the anatomy, muscles, fascia, innervations, and supporting structures involved in male continence. However, our understanding of long-term changes that occur in the pelvic floor and urethral sphincter over a period of time is more limited. Hacad et al. evaluated pelvic floor electromyography (EMG) before, at 1, 3, and 6 months following radical retropubic prostatectomy. In this small group of 38 men, 18 (47.7%) patients suffered from urinary incontinence 6 months postoperatively and surface EMG showed significant changes in fast contraction amplitude, rest amplitude following fast contraction, and in 10 second sustained contraction amplitude possibly as a result of nerve changes to the external urethral sphincter suggesting a whole new urethral sphincter functionality or condition following radical retropubic prostatectomy procedure [6]. In another elegant prospective study by Catarin et al., 44 patients were evaluated and they were able to show that pudenda-anal and pudenda-urethral reflexes were basically unchanged 6 months following nerve-sparing prostatectomy confirming unchanged sensory and motor pudendal innervations to the pelvic region. However, 34 (77.3%) of the patients demonstrated significant autonomic denervation of the membranous urethral mucosa which was associated with urinary incontinence [7].

Many experts believe that main contributing factor to urinary incontinence postprostatectomy is due to urethral sphincter incompetency [8] possibly due to multiple etiologies but mainly nerve damage [9]. In addition, bladder dysfunction and lower urinary tract symptoms (LUTS) have been attributed to indirectly affect continence in this group of patients. Changes in geometric bladder anatomy, location, inflammation, and neuroplasticity can also contribute to detrusor dysfunction following radical prostatectomy procedure.

Haga et al. used magnetic resonance imaging postprostatectomy to show urinary pooling in the urethra as a possible explanation for inducing urgency [10]. Porena et al. reviewed literature and reported a de novo detrusor overactivity of 2–77%, decreased bladder compliance in 8–39%, impaired detrusor contractility in 29–61% of patients [11]. Multiple studies in the literature have also shown an association between detrusor overactivity and urinary incontinence following radical prostatectomy [12, 13]. Urodynamic evaluation immediately following RARP in 87 patients showed a decrease in cystometric capacity (from 341 to 250 ml) and a decrease in maximal urethral closure pressure (from 84.6 to 35.6 cmH$_2$O). In addition, 75 (86%) of the patients demonstrated an abdominal leak point pressure of 47.7 cmH$_2$O [14]. Hammer and Huland showed significant bladder and sphincter changes after radical prostatectomy. They found decreases in bladder capacity, bladder compliance, and an increase in bladder instability [15]. However, Asnat et al. found the primary cause of postprostatectomy incontinence is sphincteric in nature, affecting 88% of men. In fact, it was the only cause of incontinence in 32.5% of men [16]. Nonetheless, detrusor instability was identified in 33.7% but was the primary cause of incontinence in only 7.2% [17]. Giannantoni et al. carried out a well-designed study involving 49 patients. They evaluated these patients just before surgery, 1 and 8 months postoperatively. These authors found detrusor overactivity was present in 55% of patients before surgery and persisted with little change in 1 and 8 months postoperatively. Furthermore, 28.6% of the patients developed hypocontractility, possibly due to transient bladder denervation at the time of surgery. Additionally, at 1 month 18.4% of the men and at 6 months 10.2% of the men had de novo and continued decrease in compliance of their bladders [18].

These data suggest there is more to postprostatectomy incontinence than just urethral competency, thus providing other target areas for intervention. So, what can we do in an adjuvant or near term fashion to get our patients continent, and to do so in as short a period of time as possible? The area of adjuvant management is checkered with anecdotal surgeon-specific notions, ideas, and surgical techniques. There are many small, nonrandomized single surgeon trials and larger, well-done trials with equivocal results. Despite the distinct lack of clearly superior results, there are things we can do that may help, and we shall review these options in this chapter. Adjuvant therapies fall into basically four categories: pharmacological, physical in the form of pelvic floor exercises, surgical (male urethral sling, artificial urinary sphincter), and investigational such as stem cells. In this chapter, we will provide detailed reviews of current literature and valuable insights into each of the above categories.

Pharmacological Intervention

Some pharmacological agents have been evaluated postprostatectomy to potentially improve overall incontinence in patients. Tolterodine, vardenafil, tadalafil, solifenacin, and duloxetine have been proposed to address the lower urinary tract dysfunction and the bladder stability and thus improve the overall continence rate.

Anticholinergic Medications

It appears that since bladder dysfunction has some role in postoperative incontinence, anticholinergics or other medications that improve overactive bladder symptoms may impact the recovery to urinary continence. Many if not most urologists use anticholinergics as a part of their postoperative incontinence regimen. However, not many controlled trials have been carried out to evaluate the benefits of these medications. Liss et al., in an early pilot study, evaluated the usefulness of solifenacin in patients undergoing Robotic Prostatectomy by a single surgeon. They hypothesized that return of continence at greater than 3 months was in large part due to detrusor overactivity and/or dysfunction. Forty men were enrolled and "appeared" to benefit [19]. This trial led to a large, multicenter randomized double-blinded study of the anticholinergic, solifenacin, in men undergoing Robotic Prostatectomy. This well-designed study had a phase-in time of from 7 to 21 days after catheter removal, to allow a washout period for those on preoperative anticholinergics and also to exclude those who achieved complete urinary control in this early period. Patients were randomized one to one to solifenacin or a placebo. Patients were also given a smart phone-like device called a PDA (Diary Pro, Invivo Data/eResearch Technology, Inc., Philadelphia, Pennsylvania) which evaluated daily pad use and drug intake. The PDA alerted patients every evening until the necessary information was entered. The primary endpoint was a time to complete urinary control at 3 months from first dose of study drug. Over 1000 patients were screened and 640 were randomized. Although there was no statistical difference in time to continence, 29 % of the solifenacin group versus 21 % of the placebo group achieved complete continence, $P=0.04$. In addition, pads per day usage in the treatment group decreased by 3.2 pads per day versus 2.9 in the controlled group, $P=0.03$. Adverse events, such as constipation, were the same for both groups but, as expected, dry mouth was more common in the treatment group, 6.1 % versus 0.6 %. Although the primary endpoint of the time to return of continence was not achieved, important secondary endpoints were. Namely, 99/313 solifenacin versus 66/309 placebo achieved continence during this 3-month study and pad usage decreased by a statistically significant margin in favor of the treatment arm. Limitations of this study include: no urodynamics testing was carried out preoperatively or postoperatively, the digital PDA used to record progress may have had an associated placebo effect, and that longer term follow-up up to 12 months was not designed in the study. Nonetheless, this study underscores potential benefits of anticholinergics in this patient population [20].

Alpha Agonists

As the bladder neck, trigone, and the membranous urethra are rich in alpha receptors, many urologists have over time used the alpha stimulating agents such as ephedrine and pseudoephedrine hydrochloride to help speed postprostatectomy incontinence recovery. The hope has been that by stimulating alpha receptors, a better closure of the bladder neck and sphincter can be achieved, resulting in greater resistance to flow and improved continence. Few clinical trials however have been carried out and reported. Furthermore, most of these drugs have a side effect profile (hypertension and CNS effects) that limits their usefulness and tolerability.

Radley et al. studied the usefulness of methoxamine, an α_1 adrenoceptor selective agonist in women with stress urinary incontinence. This small trial was a double-blinded crossover study giving the women placebo or methoxamine IV and measuring urethral pressures. Although statistical significance was not achieved, at the highest dose there was a definitive increase in maximum urethral pressure. Unfortunately, there was a significant increase in systolic blood pressure and decrease in pulse rate. Furthermore, all the subjects reported piloerection ("goose-flesh"), cold extremities, and headaches. The modest gain in urethral pressure was more that outweighed by the side effect profile [21].

In summary, alpha agonists may have a role to play, albeit a small one? Use of these drugs should be considered with care and patients need to be aware of potential toxicities and monitored accordingly.

Other Pharmaceutical Agents

Duloxetine

Duloxetine is a serotonin/norepinephrine reuptake inhibitor which has long been used in women with stress urinary incontinence. Cornu et al. in a randomized, placebo-controlled trial randomized 16 patients to 3 months of duloxetine 80 mg for three months versus 15 patients randomized to placebo. Treatment group reported significant improvement in multiple urinary questionnaires including QOL suggesting duloxetine may be a potential pharmacological intervention in postprostatectomy incontinence [22]. Filocamo et al. reported a more comprehensive and larger trial by randomizing 112 patients to PFMT plus duloxetine versus PFMT and placebo for 16 weeks. Authors reported a significantly improved in I-QOL scores and significant decrease in IEF scores. Authors also reported a discontinuation rate due to adverse events of about 15.2 % with nausea being the most common side effect [23]. Serra et al. evaluated a group of 68 men who were over a year out from radical prostatectomy and had persistent stress urinary incontinence. The median duration of treatment was approximately 6 months. Seventy-four percent of patients had a significant decrease in their International Consultation on Incontinence Questionnaire-Urinary Incontinence Short Form (ICIQ-UI-SF) and 57 % experienced a significant decrease in pad use. However, 25 % of the patients stopped taking the drug due to side effects such as mild extremity trembling, fatigue, and dry mouth [24].

Phosphodiesterase Type 5 Inhibitors (PDE5-I)

PDE5-I are known to positively affect postprostatectomy erectile dysfunctions and play an important role in potency rehabilitation postoperatively. Recent data suggests the PDE5-I can concurrently improve lower urinary tract symptoms in benign prostatic hyperplasia. Gacci et al. evaluated the role of vardenafil in continence recovery following nerve-sparing radical prostatectomy. Thirty-nine patients were randomized and double blinded to vardenafil on demand, vardenafil nightly, and placebo. Authors demonstrated that nightly vardenafil can improve postprostatectomy incontinence when compared to controls but the time to recovery is not affected by it [25]. Some investigators were also able to demonstrate a positive effect of PDE5-I on postprostatectomy incontinence [26] [27], versus others have not shown any benefit [28].

Stem Cell Therapy

In the early to mid-1990s, many investigators identified bone marrow stromal cells capable of differentiating into numerous cell lines. Caplan, in 1991, defined these as "mesenchymal" "stem cells" [29]. This definition has since been refined by the International

Society for Cell Therapy as "multipotent stromal cells" [30]. Since that discovery, well over 5000 publications have appeared in peer-reviewed literature regarding stem cells. The potential urologic opportunities for the use of these cells have also increased dramatically. The regenerative capabilities offered by stem cells have been exploited by plastic surgeons in the treatment of mastectomy defects [31] and facial defects due to trauma [32]. This regenerative option has generated much interest and enthusiasm in urologists for the potential of treating urinary incontinence and impotence.

In a comprehensive review of stem cell therapy, Damaser describes stem cells as "unique population of cells with three defining characteristics: (1) ability to self-renew; (2) multipotent differentiation potential; and (3) clonogenicity, or the ability to form clonal cell populations derived from a single stem cell." These characteristics are important in the ability of stem cells to affect repair of injured tissues, in this case the urinary rhabdosphincter [33]. Stem cells are able to be derived from a number of sources: embryonic stems cells (ESCs) and mesenchymal stem cells (MSCs), which include: placental or amniotic fluid stem cells (AFPSCs), muscle-derived stem cells (MDSC), adipose-derived stem cells (ADSC), bone-marrow-derived stem cells, and even urinary-derived stem cells (USC). The mechanism of action of stem cells is their ability to migrate to sites of acute and chronic injury where they facilitate healing. The ability of stem cells for multipotential differentiation and proliferation is felt to be the mechanism for return of urinary rhabdosphincter recovery through an increase in muscle and neuronal volume. Furthermore, it is also felt that stem cells secrete bioactive factors that have additional therapeutic benefits and are perhaps more responsible for the large, overall therapeutic effects, as stem cells do not remain long in injured tissues.

As the science of stem cells and their multipotential use in any number of diseases has improved and gained clinical traction, their use in stress urinary incontinence has grown as well. Many researchers and investigators believe that the future management of stress urinary incontinence will be by stem cell injections into the rhabdosphincter. Zhao et al., in a surgically created incontinent rat model, using adipose-derived stem cells (ADSC) with nerve growth factor, demonstrated a significant increase in rhabdosphincter muscle and ganglia and return of continence in urethral pressure profile measurements to preop levels compared to controls [34]. In another rat study by Lin et al., the animals were subjected to stretch/traumatic injury in the urethra and had their ovaries removed to simulate postmenopausal women. Animals were randomized to three groups: direct injection of ADSC to rhabdosphincter, ADSC injection into the tail vein, and a controlled group. The rats were sacrificed 4 weeks later. The results showed that 80 % of the control group had abnormal voiding function whereas only 33 % of the two treatment groups had this finding [35]. Kim et al. carried out bilateral pudendal nerve dissection and 2 weeks later had periurethral injection of muscle-derived stem cells. The results again showed that the treated animals' leak point pressures and urethral closure pressures were similar to animals subjected to sham surgery [36]. Finally, Chermansky et al., after inducing stress incontinence in female rats by midurethral cauterization, treated the animals 1 week after injury with injection of muscle-derived stem cells into the midurethra. The treated animals had significant increases in leak point pressure compared to controls, and with histologic evidence of muscle-derived stem cell integration into the urethral musculature [37].

Human trials in stress urinary incontinence have been ongoing for a number of years. Carr et al. reported on a patient population of 38 women with stress urinary incontinence who underwent muscle-derived stem cell injections into the sphincter. The women were also offered a second injection 3 months later. Ninety percent of the treated women had over a 50 % decrease in pad weight and only 50 % reported leaks. Adverse events were essentially absent [38]. Gotoh treated 11 men with persistent stress urinary incontinence 1 year after prostate surgery and demonstrated a 60 % decrease in urinary leakage volume on pads weighed by the patients. One of the 11 achieved complete return of urinary control. Functional urethral leak and urethral closing pressures were also increased compared to pretreatment levels. No adverse events were reported [39]. Currently, there is a large multicenter ongoing trial phase 3 trial in the United States with muscle-derived stem cells in women with stress urinary incontinence and a phase 1, 2 trial using muscle-derived stem cell in postprostatectomy incontinence (ClinicalTrials.gov Identifier: NCT01893138 and NCT02291432).

Although stem cells derived from any source are not yet ready for clinical use in men with stress urinary incontinence after radical retropubic prostatectomy, the future appears to hold promise. Nonetheless, ethical and regulatory issues remain of concern and may present hurdles to widespread clinical adoption [40]. The early ethical concerns surrounding the use of fetal embryonic stem cells have by and large been resolved by the development of so many other sources for multipotent stem cells. Nonetheless, the recent classification of stem cells as a "drug" places them under the purview of the FDA and now regulatory hurdles may enhance or impede the science and usefulness of these agents. Finally, the fears of the development of secondary cancers or causing early recurrences/failures of cancers if stems cells are released into the operative field to and in early functional recovery are very real. Well-structured trials need to be carried out to address these questions and the questions of which (if any) of the currently available products might be best used in men undergoing prostatectomy. Nonetheless, the future of stem cells use in our patients undergoing prostatectomy appears bright.

Conservative Management

The value of various conservative interventions to improve continence postprostatectomy is an area of debate with conflicting data. The recommended timing of when to initiate intervention and or education is not clear either. Burgio and his colleagues prospectively randomized 125 men undergoing radical prostatectomy to preoperative biofeedback-assisted behavioral training plus daily home exercises versus a usual control care (postoperative Kegel exercises). Authors found that patients with preoperative training had a significantly shorter time to continence and decreased the severity of urine leak [41].

PFPT with or Without Biofeedback

Pelvic Floor Physical Therapy refers to any technique that causes targeted and repetitive and contractile activity in specific pelvic floor muscles with the hope of training these muscle groups to actively contribute to coaptation of urethral sphincter when the intra-abdominal pressure is increased. Biofeedback also refers to auditory or visual cues to the patient during contractions to provide feedback on the quality and effectiveness of the exercise. Biofeedback can be obtained by sophisticated equipment or electromyography versus a simple feedback from the trainer by digital rectal examination. The effects of pelvic floor physical therapy on urinary incontinence recovery still stay controversial in the literature. Ribeiro et al. evaluated the long-term effects of early postoperative biofeedback-pelvic floor muscle training in 73 males who were undergoing radical prostatectomy with a 12 months follow-up. They randomized 36 patients to biofeedback-pelvic floor muscle training once a week for 3 months and a control group of 37 patients. At 12 months 25 patients in the treatment group and 21 patients in the control group were continent ($p=0.028$). In addition, it appeared that biofeedback-pelvic floor muscle therapy overall significantly improved the severity of incontinence, lower urinary tract symptoms, and quality of life of the treatment group that lasted 12 months following the procedure [42]. Different trainings and delivery method of pelvic floor muscle training (PFMT) to the patients have been evaluated and the literature has inconsistent data. For instance, Moore et al. in a multicenter randomized trial stratified 205 patients to weekly therapist-guided PFMT versus standardized verbal and written instructions and demonstrated no significant differences between groups at 8, 12, 28, and 52 weeks [43]. These data may suggest a less-intense, standard therapy may be as effective but less costly for the system. On the contrary some experts believe that intensive prolonged and early initiation of PFMT can improve continence that persists in the first 12 months [44]. A recent and comprehensive Cochrane review on eight trials showed that there is no evidence to support PFPT with or without biofeedback to be more effective than control for patients up to 12 months following radical prostatectomy [45].

Authors caution us with the significant variations in the patients, interventions, data, and outcome measures, but overall it appeared that patients' continence improved over time regardless of intervention.

Some experts have suggested and questioned that possibly initiating preoperative PFPT may improve continence outcomes [46, 47]. In a meta-analysis to evaluate preoperative intervention with PFPT, Wang et al. included five studies but reported insufficient data to report any benefit in quality of life or continence benefits with preprostatectomy PFPT [48].

Electrical Stimulation and Extracorporeal Magnetic Innervation

Data on electrical stimulation either used alone or in conjunction with behavioral therapy or physical therapy is conflicting in the literature. Electrical stimulation is thought to stimulate the striated urethral sphincter and thus increase its contractility.

The electrical stimulation to the pelvic floor can either be delivered through noninvasive anal probes or surface electrodes as Transcutaneous Electrical Nerve Stimulation (TENS) similar to the one's used in overactive bladder. Goode et al. in a prospective randomized control trial evaluated the role of biofeedback in patients with persistence urinary incontinence 12 months following surgery. Two-hundred and eight patients 1–17 years following their prostatectomy were stratified to three groups. Group one which included 8 weeks of behavioral therapy with pelvic floor muscle training; group 2 which included the behavioral therapy plus in office, dual-channel electromyography biofeedback in addition to daily home pelvic floor electrical stimulation; group 3 served as a delayed treatment group and a control group. The authors showed that 8 weeks of behavioral therapy compared to controls improved continence episodes whereas adding pelvic floor electrical stimulation did not increase the efficacy [49]. On the contrary, Yamanishi et al. used electrical stimulation in 56 men with severe postprostatectomy incontinence with all patients receiving concurrent pelvic floor muscle training preoperatively and throughout the recovery. Twenty-six patients were randomized to the treatment group and 30 to sham. Authors reported an improvement in amount of leakage, the International Consultation on Incontinence Questionnaire in the active group at 1 month but not at 12 months [50]. Early use of combination pelvic floor electrical stimulation and biofeedback has also shown to be effective in early recovery of urinary incontinence postprostatectomy [51].

Extra-corporeal magnetic innervation (ExMI) which stimulates pelvic floor contractions through using a magnetic field on a chair has also been proposed to improve stress and urge urinary incontinence [52]. In a small series with a short follow-up, Yokoyama and colleagues compared ExMI to functional electrical stimulation (FES) and found that these two therapies only offered an earlier return to urinary continence in 1 month compared to controls. However, at 6 months follow-up 24 h pad test was similar between the treatment groups and the controls [53]. Another smaller study examined penile vibratory stimulation (PVS) in 64 patients following radical prostatectomy. Authors reported 90 % continence in the treatment group and 94.7 % in the control group after 12 months demonstrating no documented benefit from using PVS [54].

Life Style Changes

Life style changes would include time voiding, fluid management, and overall changes that would promote weight loss, smoking cessation, healthy diet, and exercise. Currently, there are no strong evidence that life style changes will have a direct positive affect on postprostatectomy incontinence [45].

Acupuncture

In a small Chinese study, 109 patients were stratified to PFPT with or without electrical acupuncture. At a short follow-up of 6 weeks patients with combined PFPT and electrical acupuncture had better urinary continence outcome.

However, the results were not long lasting and both groups had similar outcomes at 16 weeks [55].

Pilates and Concentration Therapy

In hopes to improve effectiveness of PFPT, treating physicians have explored adjunctive methods to PFPT. Pilates includes stretching and core stability exercises that focus on pelvic floor, body alignment, and trunk muscles. In addition, these exercises are performed in coordination of deep breathing and focus on intra-abdominal pressures. Pedriali et al. randomized 85 patients to three groups of G1: Pilates, G2: Pilates and PFPT, G3: control group. Both treatment groups performed ten weekly sessions. Authors reported no statistically significant difference between the two treatment groups in regards to daily pad use, 24 h pad test, ICIQ-SF scores. The authors concluded that Pilates exercises can be as effective as PFPT in postprostatectomy incontinence and it may even contribute to higher continent rates when compared to controls in short term [56]. Concentration therapy is very varied among practitioner and the data can be conflicting, never the less a small Thai study compared PFPT with or without concentration therapy and reported some benefits [57]. Authors of this chapter believe that these data need to be replicated in larger randomized trials with standardized continence measurements before general recommendation or use.

Compression Devices (Penile Clamps)

External devices have long been used in urology to control the urinary leak. Penile clamps have evolved to become easier to use, disposable, and only compressing on the ventral side [58, 59]. Condom catheters have also been used in significant incontinence especially in the neurogenic bladder setting or for overnight control.

Late Intervention

Surgical interventions: Like balloon adjustable implants, bulking agents, slings, and artificial urinary sphincter (AUS) are the last resort if all other adjunctive measures fail.

Conclusion

In conclusion based on the review of the literature, there is a paucity of level 1 evidence in adjunctive measures to improve urinary continence in the early and late period following radical prostatectomy. Future prospective studies in large group of patients with longer follow-up are needed to evaluate each intervention in more detail. In addition, we need to understand the anatomical and functional changes that follow radical prostatectomy in each patient with higher degree of precision to be able to individualize our recommendations and treatments.

References

1. Gibbs CF, Johnson 2nd TM, Ouslander JG. Office management of geriatric urinary incontinence. Am J Med. 2007;120:211.
2. Kumar A, Samavedi S, Bates AS, et al. Continence outcomes of robot assisted radical prostatectomy in patients with adverse urinary continence risk factors. BJU Int. 2015;116(5):764–70.
3. Lavigueur-Blouin H, Noriega AC, Valdivieso R, et al. Predictors of early continence following robot-assisted radical prostatectomy. Can Urol Assoc J. 2015;9:93.
4. Matsushita K, Kent MT, Vickers AJ, et al. Preoperative predictive model of recovery of urinary continence after radical prostatectomy. BJU Int. 2015;116(4):577–83.
5. Holm HV, Fossa SD, Hedlund H, et al. How should continence and incontinence after radical prostatectomy be evaluated? A prospective study of patient ratings and changes with time. J Urol. 2014;192:1155.
6. Hacad CR, Glazer HI, Zambon JP, et al. Is there any change in pelvic floor electromyography during the first 6 months after radical retropubic prostatectomy? Appl Psychophysiol Biofeedback. 2015;40:9.
7. Catarin MV, Manzano GM, Nobrega JA, et al. The role of membranous urethral afferent autonomic innervation in the continence mechanism after nerve sparing radical prostatectomy: a clinical and prospective study. J Urol. 2008;180:2527.
8. Majoros A, Bach D, Keszthelyi A, et al. Urinary incontinence and voiding dysfunction after radical retropubic prostatectomy (prospective urodynamic study). Neurourol Urodyn. 2006;25:2.
9. Dubbelman YD, Bosch JL. Urethral sphincter function before and after radical prostatectomy: systematic review of the prognostic value of various assessment techniques. Neurourol Urodyn. 2013;32:957.
10. Haga N, Ogawa S, Yabe M, et al. Association between postoperative pelvic anatomic features on magnetic resonance imaging and lower tract urinary symptoms after radical prostatectomy. Urology. 2014;84:642.
11. Porena M, Mearini E, Mearini L, et al. Voiding dysfunction after radical retropubic prostatectomy: more than external urethral sphincter deficiency. Eur Urol. 2007;52:38.
12. Rodriguez Jr E, Skarecky DW, Ahlering TE. Post-robotic prostatectomy urinary continence: characterization of perfect continence versus occasional dribbling in pad-free men. Urology. 2006;67:785.
13. Dubbelman Y, Groen J, Wildhagen M, et al. Quantification of changes in detrusor function and pressure-flow parameters after radical prostatectomy: relation to postoperative continence status and the impact of intensity of pelvic floor muscle exercises. Neurourol Urodyn. 2012;31:637.
14. Kadono Y, Ueno S, Yaegashi H, et al. Urodynamic evaluation before and immediately after robot-assisted radical prostatectomy. Urology. 2014;84:106.
15. Hammerer P, Huland H. Urodynamic evaluation of changes in urinary control after radical retropubic prostatectomy. J Urol. 1997;157:233.
16. Groutz A, Blaivas JG, Chaikin DC, et al. The pathophysiology of post-radical prostatectomy incontinence: a clinical and video urodynamic study. J Urol. 2000;163:1767.
17. Loughlin KR, Prasad MM. Post-prostatectomy urinary incontinence: a confluence of 3 factors. J Urol. 2010;183:871.
18. Giannantoni A, Mearini E, Di Stasi SM, et al. Assessment of bladder and urethral sphincter function before and after radical retropubic prostatectomy. J Urol. 2004;171:1563.
19. Liss MA, Morales B, Skarecky D, et al. Phase 1 clinical trial of vesicare (solifenacin) in the treatment of urinary incontinence after radical prostatectomy. J Endourol. 2014;28:1241.

20. Bianco FJ, Albala DM, Belkoff LH, et al. A randomized, double-blind, solifenacin succinate versus placebo control, phase 4, multicenter study evaluating urinary continence after robotic assisted radical prostatectomy. J Urol. 2015;193:1305.

21. Radley SC, Chapple CR, Bryan NP, et al. Effect of methoxamine on maximum urethral pressure in women with genuine stress incontinence: a placebo-controlled, double-blind crossover study. Neurourol Urodyn. 2001;20:43.

22. Cornu JN, Merlet B, Ciofu C, et al. Duloxetine for mild to moderate postprostatectomy incontinence: preliminary results of a randomised, placebo-controlled trial. Eur Urol. 2011;59:148.

23. Filocamo MT, Li Marzi V, Del Popolo G, et al. Pharmacologic treatment in postprostatectomy stress urinary incontinence. Eur Urol. 2007;51:1559.

24. Collado Serra A, Rubio-Briones J, Puyol Payas M, et al. Postprostatectomy established stress urinary incontinence treated with duloxetine. Urology. 2011;78:261.

25. Gacci M, Ierardi A, Rose AD, et al. Vardenafil can improve continence recovery after bilateral nerve sparing prostatectomy: results of a randomized, double blind, placebo-controlled pilot study. J Sex Med. 2010;7:234.

26. Gandaglia G, Albersen M, Suardi N, et al. Postoperative phosphodiesterase type 5 inhibitor administration increases the rate of urinary continence recovery after bilateral nerve-sparing radical prostatectomy. Int J Urol. 2013;20:413.

27. Hubanks JM, Umbreit EC, Karnes RJ, et al. Open radical retropubic prostatectomy using high anterior release of the levator fascia and constant haptic feedback in bilateral neurovascular bundle preservation plus early postoperative phosphodiesterase type 5 inhibition: a contemporary series. Eur Urol. 2012;61:878.

28. Canat L, Guner B, Gurbuz C, et al. Effects of three-times-per-week versus on-demand tadalafil treatment on erectile function and continence recovery following bilateral nerve sparing radical prostatectomy: results of a prospective, randomized, and single-center study. Kaohsiung J Med Sci. 2015;31:90.

29. Caplan AI. Mesenchymal stem cells. J Orthop Res. 1991;9:641.

30. Dominici M, Le Blanc K, Mueller I, et al. Minimal criteria for defining multipotent mesenchymal stromal cells. The International Society for Cellular Therapy position statement. Cytotherapy. 2006;8:315.

31. Matsumoto D, Sato K, Gonda K, et al. Cell-assisted lipotransfer: supportive use of human adipose-derived cells for soft tissue augmentation with lipoinjection. Tissue Eng. 2006;12:3375.

32. Yoshimura K, Sato K, Aoi N, et al. Cell-assisted lipotransfer for facial lipoatrophy: efficacy of clinical use of adipose-derived stem cells. Dermatol Surg. 2008;34:1178.

33. Goldman HB, Sievert KD, Damaser MS. Will we ever use stem cells for the treatment of SUI? ICI-RS 2011. Neurourol Urodyn. 2012;31:386.

34. Zhao W, Zhang C, Jin C, et al. Periurethral injection of autologous adipose-derived stem cells with controlled-release nerve growth factor for the treatment of stress urinary incontinence in a rat model. Eur Urol. 2011;59:155.

35. Lin G, Wang G, Banie L, et al. Treatment of stress urinary incontinence with adipose tissue-derived stem cells. Cytotherapy. 2010;12:88.

36. Kim SO, Na HS, Kwon D, et al. Bone-marrow-derived mesenchymal stem cell transplantation enhances closing pressure and leak point pressure in a female urinary incontinence rat model. Urol Int. 2011;86:110.

37. Chermansky CJ, Tarin T, Kwon DD, et al. Intraurethral muscle-derived cell injections increase leak point pressure in a rat model of intrinsic sphincter deficiency. Urology. 2004;63:780.

38. Carr LK, Steele D, Steele S, et al. 1-year follow-up of autologous muscle-derived stem cell injection pilot study to treat stress urinary incontinence. Int Urogynecol J Pelvic Floor Dysfunct. 2008;19:881.

39. Gotoh M, Yamamoto T, Kato M, et al. Regenerative treatment of male stress urinary incontinence by periurethral injection of autologous adipose-derived regenerative cells: 1-year outcomes in 11 patients. Int J Urol. 2014;21:294.

40. Edwards RG. A burgeoning science of embryological genetics demands a modern ethics. Reprod Biomed Online. 2007;15 Suppl 1:34.

41. Burgio KL, Goode PS, Urban DA, et al. Preoperative biofeedback assisted behavioral training to decrease post-prostatectomy incontinence: a randomized, controlled trial. J Urol. 2006;175:196.
42. Ribeiro LH, Prota C, Gomes CM, et al. Long-term effect of early postoperative pelvic floor biofeedback on continence in men undergoing radical prostatectomy: a prospective, randomized, controlled trial. J Urol. 2010;184:1034.
43. Moore KN, Valiquette L, Chetner MP, et al. Return to continence after radical retropubic prostatectomy: a randomized trial of verbal and written instructions versus therapist-directed pelvic floor muscle therapy. Urology. 2008;72:1280.
44. Manassero F, Traversi C, Ales V, et al. Contribution of early intensive prolonged pelvic floor exercises on urinary continence recovery after bladder neck-sparing radical prostatectomy: results of a prospective controlled randomized trial. Neurourol Urodyn. 2007;26:985.
45. Anderson CA, Omar MI, Campbell SE, et al. Conservative management for postprostatectomy urinary incontinence. Cochrane Database Syst Rev. 2012;1:CD001843.
46. Centemero A, Rigatti L, Giraudo D, et al. Preoperative pelvic floor muscle exercise for early continence after radical prostatectomy: a randomised controlled study. Eur Urol. 2010;57:1039.
47. Geraerts I, Van Poppel H, Devoogdt N, et al. Influence of preoperative and postoperative pelvic floor muscle training (PFMT) compared with postoperative PFMT on urinary incontinence after radical prostatectomy: a randomized controlled trial. Eur Urol. 2013;64:766.
48. Wang W, Huang QM, Liu FP, et al. Effectiveness of preoperative pelvic floor muscle training for urinary incontinence after radical prostatectomy: a meta-analysis. BMC Urol. 2014;14:99.
49. Goode PS, Burgio KL, Johnson 2nd TM, et al. Behavioral therapy with or without biofeedback and pelvic floor electrical stimulation for persistent postprostatectomy incontinence: a randomized controlled trial. JAMA. 2011;305:151.
50. Yamanishi T, Mizuno T, Watanabe M, et al. Randomized, placebo controlled study of electrical stimulation with pelvic floor muscle training for severe urinary incontinence after radical prostatectomy. J Urol. 2010;184:2007.
51. Mariotti G, Sciarra A, Gentilucci A, et al. Early recovery of urinary continence after radical prostatectomy using early pelvic floor electrical stimulation and biofeedback associated treatment. J Urol. 2009;181:1788.
52. Galloway NT, El-Galley RE, Sand PK, et al. Update on extracorporeal magnetic innervation (EXMI) therapy for stress urinary incontinence. Urology. 2000;56:82.
53. Yokoyama T, Nishiguchi J, Watanabe T, et al. Comparative study of effects of extracorporeal magnetic innervation versus electrical stimulation for urinary incontinence after radical prostatectomy. Urology. 2004;63:264.
54. Fode M, Borre M, Ohl DA, et al. Penile vibratory stimulation in the recovery of urinary continence and erectile function after nerve-sparing radical prostatectomy: a randomized, controlled trial. BJU Int. 2014;114:111.
55. Yang BS, Ye DW, Yao XD, et al. The study of electrical acupuncture stimulation therapy combined with pelvic floor muscle therapy for postprostatectomy incontinence. Zhonghua Wai Ke Za Zhi. 2010;48:1325.
56. Pedriali, F. R., Gomes, C. S., Soares, L. et al.: Is pilates as effective as conventional pelvic floor muscle exercises in the conservative treatment of post-prostatectomy urinary incontinence? A randomised controlled trial. Neurourol Urodyn 2015. doi:10.1002/nau.22761
57. Kongtragul J, Tukhanon W, Tudpudsa P, et al. Effects of adding concentration therapy to Kegel exercise to improve continence after radical prostatectomy, randomized control. J Med Assoc Thai. 2014;97:513.
58. Baumrucker GO. A new male incontinence clamp. J Urol. 1979;121:201.
59. Fowler Jr FJ, Barry MJ, Lu-Yao G, et al. Patient-reported complications and follow-up treatment after radical prostatectomy. The national medicare experience: 1988–1990 (updated June 1993). Urology. 1993;42:622.

Chapter 9
Adjunctive Measures and New Therapies to Optimize Early Return of Erectile Function

Nizar Boudiab, Usama Khater, Shirin Razdan, and Sanjay Razdan

Introduction

Even after the advent of nerve-sparing procedure a significant percent of patients still develop erectile dysfunction after radical prostatectomy [1]. Modifications in the surgical technique of robotic radical prostatectomy have aimed not only to spare the cavernous nerve but also to minimize any potential harm done from manipulation, traction, or thermal injury of the nerves in addition to sparing the microcirculation surrounding the prostate. The adjunctive measures to optimize early return of erectile function can be subdivided into intraoperative measures designed to optimize nerve preservation and minimize injury to the neurovascular structures surrounding the prostate, and postoperative penile rehabilitation to facilitate early return of erectile function.

Electronic supplementary material The online version of this chapter (doi:10.1007/978-3-319-39448-0_9) contains supplementary material, which is available to authorized users.

N. Boudiab, M.D. • U. Khater, M.D. • S. Razdan, M.D., M.Ch. (✉)
International Robotic Prostatectomy Institute, Urology Center of Excellence at Jackson South Hospital, Deering Medical Plaza, 9380 SW 150th Street, Suite 200, Miami, FL 33176, USA

S. Razdan, B.S.
University of Miami Miller School of Medicine, Miami, FL, USA
e-mail: urodoc96@aol.com

© Springer International Publishing Switzerland 2016
S. Razdan (ed.), *Urinary Continence and Sexual Function After Robotic Radical Prostatectomy*, DOI 10.1007/978-3-319-39448-0_9

Intraoperative Measures to Optimize Early Return of Erectile Function

1. *Judicious use of thermal energy and clipless nerve preservation*: We have been using thermal energy with a combination of bipolar cautery, smart bipolar (PK dissector), and monopolar cautery in a judicious manner during our nerve-sparing robotic-assisted radical prostatectomies (RALP) with no detrimental effect on return of erectile function. Our experience in over 1000 patients (unpublished data) with this modified technique of judicious use of thermal energy has obviated the need for hemolock clips in the majority of patients essentially making the procedure "clipless" (see video 9.1).

   *This modification also ensures **consistency** in the procedure without the vagaries of the technical skill set of a bedside assistant in placing hemolock clips in a very delicate position. The surgeon, being solely responsible for controlling the prostatic pedicle and dissecting the NVB, has more control of this very critical portion of the procedure. This allows greater reproducibility without the variable of the ability of a bedside assistant. In our experience this modification has improved outcomes in terms of erectile function and reduced the complications associated with use of hemolock clips* (see video 9.2).

2. *Human amniotic membrane allograft nerve wrap*: Dehydrated Human Amniotic Membrane (dHAM) derived from the inner layer of the placenta of pregnant women is rich in cytokines and regenerative growth factors. Human amniotic membrane usage has been well established in a wide variety of reconstructive and regenerative clinical scenarios. Current clinical application includes management of burns, chronic ulcers, dural defects, intra-abdominal adhesions, peritoneal reconstruction, genital reconstruction, hip arthroplasty, tendon repair, nerve repair, microvascular reconstruction, corneal repair, intra-oral reconstruction, and reconstruction of the nasal lining and tympanic membrane [2, 3]. Amniotic epithelial and mesenchymal cells have been shown to contain a variety of regulatory mediators that result in promotion of cellular proliferation, differentiation and epithelialization and the inhibition of fibrosis, immune rejection, inflammation, and bacterial invasion. Bilateral neurovascular bundle (NVB) preservation has been shown to be a positive indicator of return of potency post radical prostatectomy. However there are factors negatively impact the early return of erectile function. These factors include thermal injury, inflammatory response, traction injury, and scar tissue formation [4]. Minimizing these negative effects on nerve preservation and regeneration is one of the prime goals of a well done robotic radical prostatectomy [5].

   At our International Robotic Prostatectomy Institute we first used dHAM in a pilot study in 2012. Encouraged by the results we conducted a study to evaluate the effect of dHAM (Amniofix, MiMedx, Marietta, GA) on the return of erectile function in patients undergoing robotic radical prostatectomy. *To the best of our knowledge this was the first retrospective study in the world describing the technique and outcomes of the use of dHAM in patients undergoing bilateral nerve-sparing robotic radical prostatectomy.* The results were presented at the World

Congress of Endourology in August 2014. The study included two groups of patients: group 1 had 38 patients who underwent RALP without application of dHAM and group 2 had 22 patients who underwent RALP with use of dHAM. Both groups were comparable with respect to age, comorbidities, Gleason score, preop PSA, and SHIM score. Patients in both dHAM nerve wrap group and control group underwent standard robot-assisted laparoscopic radical prostatectomy (RALP) with maximal bilateral nerve preservation. Bilateral intrafascial neurovascular bundle preservation using our modified (clipless) athermal technique with point cauterization as required was utilized in all patients. In Group 2, before vesicourethral anastomosis, a 4×6 cm dHAM strip was applied over bilateral neurovascular bundles through an assistant port. Based on the width and configuration of the preserved NVB the dHAM (Figs. 9.1 and 9.2) was used either as a single wrap covering the bundles or split in two and used as individual wraps over the NVBs (see video 9.3).

In the follow-up period, both groups received 5 mg tadalafil daily. Data regarding erectile function was prospectively collected using the SHIM questionnaire during follow-up visits. At the 3-month follow-up visit, 42.1 % of patients in the control group had erections and 21 % had a SHIM ≥16 (mean 7.65, SD 7.19). Whereas in the dHAM group more than 90.9 % had erections and 77.3 % had a SHIM ≥16 (mean 17.32, SD 5.65), which was significantly higher. At the 6 month follow-up visit, the trend was maintained with higher erectile function in the dHAM group. In the control group, the number of persons achieving erections slightly improved to 52.6 %. The mean SHIM score was 11.02 (SD 8.07). In the dHAM group all except one patient had achieved erections with a SHIM ≥16.

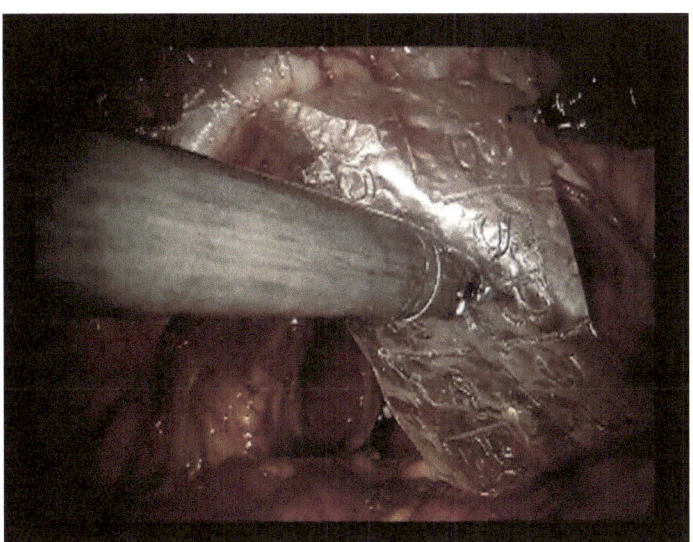

Fig. 9.1 Single dHAM wrap for NVB

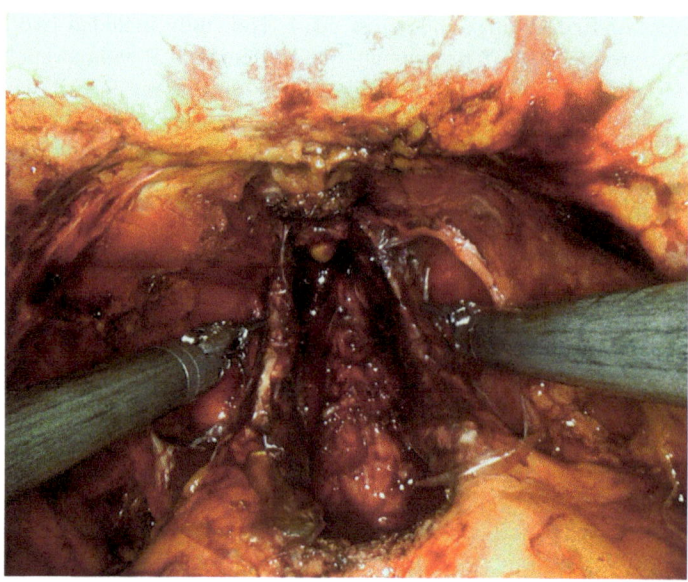

Fig. 9.2 Individual dHAM wraps for NVB

The study showed that use of dHAM as a nerve wrap over the preserved NVBs during RALP has a significant impact on early recovery of erectile function. We feel that use of dHAM is a useful adjunct to a meticulous NVB preservation during robotic radical prostatectomy and most likely is instrumental in reducing the inflammatory response and traction injuries which are often unavoidable even in the hands of the most experienced surgeons.

Postoperative Measures to Optimize Early Return of Erectile Function

Despite the nerve-sparing technique of radical prostatectomy, erectile dysfunction can be a complication as the cavernous nerve is not a major nerve branch that can easily be identified and separated from the prostate. On the contrary, it ramifies into a plexus of small nerves that are adherent to the prostatic capsule. However, even with preservation of the cavernous nerve, there is a temporary and reversible period of erectile impairment after the surgery which is caused by the manipulation, trauma, or inflammatory changes of the nerve plexus. These manipulations cause neuropraxia which is a temporary block of nerve transmission despite an anatomical intact nerve fiber. That temporary nerve dysfunction leads to structural changes in the penile tissue. This is linked to the finding that oxygen tension is 25–43 mmHg in the flaccid penis, while it increases to about 100 mmHg in the erect state [6].

During the period of neuropraxia, the penile tissue is in constant state of low oxygen supply, which may lead to smooth muscle apoptosis and fibrosis [7]. This disrupts the veno-occlusive mechanism, which is crucial in normal erectile function and structural damage could be the cause of long term ED after nerve-sparing prostatectomy [8, 9].

Better understanding of the pathophysiology of erectile dysfunction after RP erectile or penile rehabilitation has emerged.

Penile Rehabilitation

The concept of penile rehabilitation is to start erectile dysfunction treatment at the time of reversible neuropraxia of the cavernous nerve, before irreversible changes that result in permanent erectile dysfunction take place. The idea was first developed by Montorsi et al., who first reported the positive effect of intracorporeal alprostadil treatment after radical prostatectomy. Since then, many studies on the subject have been published over the past decade [10].

Penile rehabilitation consists of using medications, devices, and procedures to help recover erectile function after radical prostatectomy. Numerous studies have shown that patients who underwent penile rehabilitation had a faster recovery of their erectile function [11–15]. PDE5 inhibitors, intraurethral medications, intracavernosal injections, vacuum erection devices, and penile prostheses are the main treatments used for penile rehabilitation following radical prostatectomy.

These treatment modalities are used for treating erectile dysfunction as well as penile rehabilitation. However, beyond their conventional management of erectile dysfunction, when used for penile rehabilitation, their main purpose is to help restoring a natural level of erectile function after surgery with the objective of achieving satisfactory performance in sexual activity, without the need for further medical assistance of erectile aids.

It has been reported that 87 % of physicians use these treatments in some form for penile rehabilitation [16]. However, despite their common use, until now, there has not been any standardized regimen or specific recommendations or guidelines for an optimal penile rehabilitation strategy. Therefore, these therapies are applied differently in various clinical practice patterns, according to physicians' and patients' preferences.

Even with the lack of guidelines, a tendency of advancing in treatment options successively from lesser to greater invasiveness has been commonly practiced in the management of penile rehabilitation. In general, oral PDE5 inhibitors, with or without a VED, are considered a first-line treatment option.

Second-line therapies such as intracavernosal injections or intraurethral injections of vasoactive agents and VEDs are usually offered to patients who had a non-nerve-sparing radical prostatectomy (NNSRP) or to patients who did not show satisfactory results with oral PDE5 inhibitors. A penile implant is considered a third-line treatment for patients who fail to respond to medical therapies.

With any penile rehabilitation regimen, it has been emphasized to start treatment as soon as possible after the surgery in order to prevent smooth muscle atrophy and fibrotic changes in the corpora cavernosa [11, 17–23].

This chapter provides a review of conventional treatment modalities of erectile dysfunction and their applicability into rehabilitative programs in radical prostatectomy patients, as well as an insight into new technological advances and therapeutic approaches in this field.

Phosphodiesterase Type 5 Inhibitors

Since their introduction in 1998, PDE5 inhibitors have become the main treatment option for erectile dysfunction. This is because of their high safety profile, simple oral intake, and high efficacy. By competitively binding to the catalytic site of PDE5, which is the enzyme responsible for breakdown of cGMP to 5′-guanosine monophosphate (GMP), PDE 5 inhibitors induce an accumulation of cGMP in the smooth muscle cells of the corpus cavernosum, causing relaxation of the smooth muscle, an increase in arterial blood flow, and penile tumescence. This mechanism is potentiated by nitric oxide production, which is stimulated by cavernous nerves. Therefore, the mechanism of action of PDE5 inhibitors depends on a preserved cavernosal nerve function. However, one study showed the efficacy of PDE5 inhibitors treatment even in men who had undergone non-nerve-sparing radical prostatectomy, highlighting the role of non-neuronal stimulation of nitric oxide production on penile erection [24]. Although the efficacy of PDE5 inhibitors in treating erectile dysfunction has been established, their role in penile rehabilitation programs remains controversial. Multiple animal studies with cavernous nerve injury mimicking the conditions of radical prostatectomy have demonstrated that PDE5 inhibitors can prevent fibrosis and apoptotic changes in animal models, which is suggestive of a rehabilitative efficacy of PDE5 inhibitors. In contrast to multiple controlled trials designed to evaluate PDE5 inhibitors for ED treatment, a limited number of controlled trials have investigated PDE5 inhibitors in rehabilitative context.

In a prospective, double-blind, randomized controlled trial (RCT) that looked into the use of sildenafil citrate after bilateral nerve-sparing radical prostatectomy Padma-Nathan and colleagues, showed that nightly administration of sildenafil citrate beginning 4 weeks after surgery, for 36 weeks, resulted in significantly higher IIEF scores as compared to the placebo group. A dose-dependent improvement in nocturnal penile tumescence and rigidity was noted. Despite a low number of patients enrolled and other limitations, this study showed the beneficial effect of Sildenafil in penile rehabilitation after prostatectomy [14]. In a further randomized controlled trial, Mulhall and colleagues investigated the effectiveness of a newly approved PDE5 inhibitor, avanafil, in a rehabilitative regimen in prostatectomy patients. The study showed that, in patients with post-radical prostatectomy erectile dysfunction, 12 weeks of "on demand" treatment with avanafil, showed a significant increase in IIEF- EF scores, as compared to placebo, proving its benefit in penile rehabilitation after surgery [15]. In the REINVENT (Recovery of Erections: Intervention with vardenafil Early Nightly Therapy) trial conducted by Montorsi and colleagues, patients were randomized into taking nightly vardenafil hydrochloride, on-demand vardenafil hydrochloride, or placebo for 9 months, starting within 1 month after nerve-sparing radical prostatectomy. This trial did not show any significant differences in improving erectile function and sexual intercourse completion rates between the treatment groups and placebo after the 8-week washout period. Similarly, in the open-label phase of this trial, no advantage of the treatment arm over placebo was shown [25].

The REACT trial is another randomized controlled trial by Montorsi and colleagues, which compared the efficacy of daily tadalafil, on demand tadalafil, and a placebo in patients with nerve-sparing radical prostatectomy. Similarly to the REINVENT trial, there was no significant difference in erectile function recovery between the three groups after the washout period. However, this trial looked also into the effect of treatment on reducing the loss of penile length [26].

It was shown that, at 9 months of treatment, patients in the daily tadalafil group had significantly less shrinkage of penile length compared to the other groups, which is suggestive of a protective role of PDE5 inhibitors against neuropraxia-induced structural changes after prostatectomy.

Along with some methodologic and interpretative concerns, the conflicting results of these studies leave a main controversy about the role and effectiveness of PDE5 inhibitors in erectile rehabilitation after radical prostatectomy. Despite this ongoing controversy, penile rehabilitation continues to be commonly used in everyday clinical practice, and supportive animal and human studies continue to emerge.

A recent study by Natali and colleagues, where a retrospective analysis on the effect of no treatment, on demand PDE5 inhibitors treatment, and regimented rehabilitative PDE5 inhibitors treatment on erectile function of patients post nerve-sparing radical prostatectomy, showed that oral treatment with PDE5-Is was superior to no therapy. However, the consecutive regimented program did not appear to be superior to on-demand therapy [27].

While PDE5 inhibitors' role in penile rehabilitation is yet to be determined, new PDE5 inhibitors drugs have been developed.

Avanafil

In addition to sildenafil, tadalafil, and vardenafil, the US FDA has recently approved avanafil, a highly selective PDE5 inhibitor, as an oral medication for the treatment of ED. Improvement in erectile function has been superior to placebo with all three available doses (50,100, or 200 mg) of the drug. Due to a unique chemical structure, avanafil displays a high selectivity, fast onset of action (20–40 min after drug administration) and a favorable side-effect profile, with no restrictions on food or alcohol consumption, and little impact on heart rate and systolic blood pressure when co-administered with nitrates [28]. Avanafil has been reported to treat severe cases of erectile dysfunction in patients who did not respond to other oral PDE5 inhibitors. Also avanafil has been shown effective in treating erectile dysfunction in post-nerve-sparing radical prostatectomy and diabetic patients. The effectiveness of avanafil has been reported in several studies, the most notable was the previously mentioned randomized controlled trial by Mulhall and colleagues on penile rehabilitation with 100 and 200 mg on demand avanafil treatment in post-prostatectomy patients [15].

Mirodenafil

Mirodenfil is another newly developed and marketed oral PDE5 inhibitor in South Korea that is showing a high efficacy in treating erectile dysfunction. In animal studies, Mirodenafil improved erectile function and increased nitrous oxide synthase (NOS) and cGMP in bilateral nerve-injured rats. In a multicenter, randomized, double-blind, placebo-controlled trial in a representative population of Korean men, a 12-week "on demand" treatment with Mirodenafil in fixed doses of 50 or 100 mg, has significantly improved erectile function and was well tolerated. It has been shown *effective* in treating erectile dysfunction of different causes and severities, including diabetic patients and patients on concomitant antihypertensive medications [29].

Lodenafil

Lodenafil is another drug option under development in Brazil. In crude extracts from human platelets, Lodenafil carbonate was more potent than Sildenafil in inhibiting the hydrolysis of cyclic GMP [30]. In a Phase III, randomized, double-blind, placebo-controlled clinical trial, 40 or 80 mg Lodenafil carbonate treatment significantly improved all domain scores of the IIEF and SEP questions 2 and 3 in patients with different degrees of erectile dysfunction. Mild side effects were reported including headache, rhinitis, flushing, visual color disorders, and dyspepsia.

Udenafil

Udenafil is currently only available in South Korea and registered under the name Zydena. In a randomized, placebo-controlled clinical trial, a 12 week treatment with udenafil at the dose of 100 mg improved erectile function in patients with mild-to-severe erectile dysfunction.

Udenafil has a sustained effect for 12 h after a single dose. There is also evidence of its role in treating erectile dysfunction caused by hypercholesterolemia and endothelial dysfunction secondary to diabetes mellitus.

The rapidly growing experience with PDE5 inhibitors is paralleled with the emergence of new, highly selective drugs within this class of compounds. While their effectiveness in penile rehabilitation is not confirmed, basic and clinical research in this field continue to provide support of their restorative role in managing erectile dysfunction in post-prostatectomy patients.

Prostaglandin E1 Therapy

Intraurethral Suppository: Alprostadil

Intraurethral Alprostadil (IUA), also known as Medicated Urethral System for Erections (MUSE), is a PGE1 analog administered as an intraurethral suppository. Its mechanism of action involves increasing cyclic adenosine $3',5'$-monophosphate (cAMP) and subsequently promoting blood flow and oxygenation of the corpora cavernosa. As it works locally through the urethra on erectile tissue [31, 32], its most common side-effect is urethral burning and penile pain. However, hypotension, syncope, and vaginal irritation in the partner have also been reported [33]. IUA is considered a second line treatment for erectile dysfunction. It is a valid alternative for patients who do not respond to oral therapy, and it is more readily tolerated than intracavernous injections. However, urethral administration is a semi-invasive approach and is considered a major drawback for many patients as compared to oral therapy. Studies have shown that early intraurethral Alprostadil therapy following radical prostatectomy is associated with improvements in IIEF scores, increased frequency of sexual activity, and increased incidence of natural erections sufficient for intercourse [34].

A prospective randomized trial that compared intraurethral Alprostadil to oral PDE5-I (sildenafil citrate) after bilateral nerve-sparing radical prostatectomy showed an earlier return of EF with both forms of treatment based on IIEF-EF Domain scores [32]. No statistically significant differences in the IIEF erectile function domain and intercourse success rates were observed between the two therapies at 1 year after surgery. It has been concluded that the return of EF with nightly Sildenafil citrate and intraurethral Alprostadil treatment appears to be similar within the first year after surgery. However, a statistically significant difference in favor of IUA was noticed at 6 months. This difference might be due to the different mechanisms of action of these two therapeutic modalities. IUA works locally, does not require an intact nerve supply, and improves sexual function irrespective of neuropraxia. On the other hand, PDE5 inhibitors require an intact nerve supply to have a beneficial effect on sexual function, and therefore, are not effective during the period of neuropraxia. Limitations of the study were high attrition rates (30 % for intraurethral pharmacotherapy, 19 % for oral pharmacotherapy) and lack of a control group.

In a previous non-randomized study that compared the effect of early intraurethral Alprostadil treatment for 6 months versus no treatment after bilateral nerve-sparing radical prostatectomy patients showed better erectile function recovery in the treatment group [34].

Overall, IUA has been proven beneficial in the management of erectile dysfunction; however, its use as a salvage treatment for erectile dysfunction refractory to oral therapy has been suggested but not proved. Also, IUA benefit in the context of penile rehabilitation is still unclear.

Previous studies were limited by a small number of subjects enrolled, high attrition rates, and other methodological drawbacks. Quality randomized controlled trials are needed to prove its effectiveness in penile rehabilitation after radical prostatectomy.

Intracavernosal Injection

Since the 1980s, intracavernosal injection (ICI) of vasoactive substances has been used in the management of erectile dysfunction. The injection consists of alprostadil (a synthetic prostaglandin E1 derivative) either alone or in combination with other vasoactive agents such as papaverine or phentolamine. Prostaglandin E1 induces smooth muscle relaxation through an NO independent pathway, by activating adenylyl cyclase (AC) and the cleavage of ATP into cAMP. Phentolamine is an α-blocker which also causes smooth muscle relaxation, and papaverine is a nonspecific phosphodiesterase inhibitor that increases both cAMP and cGMP in the corpora cavernosa. The combination of the three agents is additive and results in smooth muscle relaxation, increasing blood flow to the penis and causing an erection. This form of therapy is considered an effective treatment for ED. It is safe, has a rapid onset of action, and can be a successful treatment of various forms of erectile dysfunction [35]. ICI is a second line treatment option of ED patients who did not respond or tolerate oral PDE5 inhibitors, or patients who had a non-nerve-sparing radical prostatectomy. However, the discomfort and pain caused by penile injections affect patients' compliance with the treatment.

A series by Claro and colleagues demonstrated that patients who failed oral or intraurethral treatment for ED had good results with ICIs triple therapy [36]. Also, ICI was the first ED treatment to be studied in a penile rehabilitation context. The study was conducted by Montorsi and colleagues in 1997 [10] who compared erectile function recovery 6 months after nerve-sparing radical prostatectomy in patients who received Alprostadil ICIs postoperatively versus patients who received no treatment. The study showed a significantly higher recovery of spontaneous erection in the treatment group. Another study by Nandipati and colleagues has also suggested a potential benefit of ICI pharmacotherapy for penile rehabilitation. However, the uncontrolled, non-randomized study design may have biased the results [11].

The time to start ICI therapy was investigated by Gontero and colleagues, who evaluated patients who underwent a non-nerve-sparing radical prostatectomy, and received prostaglandin E1 injections at 1, 2–3, 4–6, and 7–12 months postoperatively [37]. The study showed that patients who received ICI within the first 3 months after radical prostatectomy achieved an erection sufficient who underwent a non-nerve-sparing radical prostatectomy, and received prostaglandin E1 injections at 1, 2–3, 4–6, and 7–12 months postoperatively [37]. The study showed that patients who received ICI within the first 3 months after radical prostatectomy achieved an erection sufficient for sexual intercourse; after that period of time, the chances of an acceptable response to Alprostadil decreased progressively with the time from the surgery.

In a further study, Mulhall and colleagues compared the effect of early versus late initiation of penile rehabilitation on erectile function [38]. They showed that an early treatment (2 months) was associated with a better erectile function outcome.

Although studies have demonstrated that erectile function improves with the early and regular use of Alprostadil ICI alone or combined with other vasoactive substances, it is not known how long the treatment should be continued in penile rehabilitation before the maximal effect is reached. Yiou and colleagues addressed this question, and showed, in a recent study that continuing Alprostadil injection after 1 year does not improve spontaneous erections [39].

Vacuum Erection Devices

The Vacuum Erection Device (VED) creates a negative pressure through a vacuum effect to draw blood into the penis, which results in an artificial erection. VED was approved by the FDA in 1982 [40, 41] Although initial studies demonstrated the effectiveness and safety profile of VED, it was not until the adoption of the penile rehabilitation concept by urologists and VEDs proven benefits in animal studies that caused its frequent use in penile rehabilitative regimens in recent years. By improving blood flow to the penis, VED was shown to reduce tissue hypoxia, smooth muscle apoptosis, and fibrotic changes of the corpora cavernosa in animal models [42–45]. The VED device contains a constriction ring that can be placed at the base of the penis in order to prevent blood outflow and maintain an erection for sexual intercourse. However, the constriction ring is not recommended for the purpose of penile rehabilitation [46, 47].

VED can be used for various causes of erectile dysfunction, and unlike many other treatments, its mechanism of action is independent of the neural pathway, therefore it's not affected by transient neuropraxia after radical prostatectomy. Furthermore, VED retains high efficacy rates in penile rehabilitation after radical prostatectomy whether nerve-sparing was performed or not. A 52 % response rate has been reported following non-nerve-sparing prostatectomy [48].

In one study, early, continuous VED use 1 month after nerve-sparing radical prostatectomy was compared to a late, on demand treatment, started at 6 months after the surgery. The early, continuous treatment group showed better erectile function and preservation of penile length at 3 months and 6 months. However,

9.5 months after the surgery, there was no significant difference in erectile function and penile length between the two groups [19].

In another prospective randomized study, where 109 patients were randomized to a daily vacuum erection device use versus observation alone, at 9 months follow-up, early VED use resulted in a lower chance of penile shrinkage, better erectile function outcome with an earlier sexual intercourse, better spousal satisfaction as well as earlier return of natural erections [18]. Furthermore, the combination of a PDE5 inhibitor (sildenafil) and VED in a subgroup of patients from the same study who were not satisfied by VED use alone, lead to superior results with significant improvements in each domain of the IIEF-5 score. Other studies have also demonstrated a better erectile function with the combination of VED and PDE5 inhibitors as compared to each mono therapy alone [49–51].

In a further study, a retrospective review of 203 patients who underwent bilateral nerve-sparing radical prostatectomy showed an earlier recovery of erectile function in patients who received PDE5 inhibitors mono therapy or in patients who received a combination of PDE5 inhibitors and VED, but not in patients who received VED mono therapy or in patients who had no treatment [52]. The Evidence for VED as a complementary therapy to PDE5 is promising, as they both work through different pathways. VED induces erection independently of neural pathway regeneration, and therefore, can reverse the detrimental effects of neuropraxia before PDE5 inhibitors or other neural pathway-dependent treatments can exert their effect on penile rehabilitation.

Overall, VED is noninvasive, cost-effective, safe to use in combination with other treatment modalities, and has shown positive results for penile rehabilitation, improvement in sexual function, and preservation of penile length. It has been suggested as a first-line option for postsurgical erectile dysfunction [41] especially for patients who have undergone non-nerve-sparing radical prostatectomy. However, it is mostly recommended in combination with PDE5 inhibitors since there is little justification for its use as a mono therapy for post-radical prostatectomy patients, and its combination with PDE5 inhibitors is promising.

Penile Prosthesis Implants

Penile prosthesis is the most definitive surgical treatment for ED refractory to other medical therapies. It maintains sexual function and prevents loss of penile length. It is considered a third-line treatment option for penile rehabilitation after all other treatment options have failed [53]. There are two types of penile implants: semirigid and inflatable devices. The inflatable device provides a more natural experience as it can be turned flaccid when not in use.

A new penile implant device has been developed. It consists of a cannula inserted into the corpora and a scrotal reservoir containing a vasoactive drug (sodium nitroprusside) [54, 55]. Erection occurs after squeezing the scrotal reservoir to deliver a certain amount of sodium nitroprusside into the cannula and subsequently into the corpora cavernosa. Refilling the reservoir can be done by direct injection of sodium nitroprusside through the scrotal skin. Further investigation is needed to establish the safety of this device, especially since a potential rupture of the scrotal reservoir (intercourse, trauma, infection) would result in systemic release of sodium nitroprusside and could be fatal. Another implant is under development. It is a device that imitates a physiologic erection without the use of pumps or reservoirs. It changes from flaccid to erect through application of heat [56].

Temporal Calcium Sulfate Penile Cast

Temporal calcium sulfate (CaSO4) penile cast is an innovative salvage therapy for patients with penile prosthesis infection [57]. The penile prosthesis infection rate is 2 %. When infection occurs, an urgent removal of the prosthesis in required in addition to antibiotic irrigation of the corpora cavernosa. The use of a temporal intracorporeal antibiotic cast composed of synthetic high purity CaSO4 has a dual benefit: first, it provides continuous antibiotic/antifungal medication after penile prosthesis removal, and second, the cast maintains phallic length during healing and reduces corporal fibrosis. It self-absorbs after approximately 4–6 weeks, and a new prosthesis is implanted after cast resorption. Further research is needed before adoption of this technique as a salvage treatment for penile prosthesis.

Nanotechnology

The application of nanotechnology in erectile dysfunction treatment is done through the topical use of nanoparticles containing erectogenic agents on the glans penis and penile shaft. Due to their small size and biochemical characteristics, the nanoparticles allow transdermal delivery of these erectogenic agents to the corpora cavernosa to achieve tumescence.

Prior to nanoparticle therapy, topical erectile dysfunction treatments weren't successful; this was mainly due to an anatomic barrier caused by the penile skin and tunica albuginea that blocks medications from reaching corporal tissue [58, 59] Healthy skin can block substances as small as 100 nm; nanoparticles are approximately 10 nm in diameter, comparable in size or often smaller than viruses, which allows them to overcome the epidermal barrier. However, whether or not the nanoparticles penetrate the tunica albuginea and the exact route of entry into the cavernosal bodies has not been established yet.

Nanoparticles provide excellent matrices for encapsulating various organic and inorganic compounds, including many biologically active materials, as well as existing and new pharmaceutical agents that can be applied therapeutically [60–64].

A study conducted by Han and colleagues showed improved erectile function in rats treated with nanoparticles encapsulating three different erectogenic agents (tadalafil, sialorphin, and NO) [65].

NO is known to reduce corporal smooth muscle tissue tone, a key factor in the physiology of erectile function. However, previous to the development of nanoparticles, its delivery to the corpora cavernous was not applicable. Sialorphin is a peptide used in animal models as an intracorporeal injection to improve erectile function [66]. The study showed improved erectile function, as compared to placebo. Of the three agents used the NO nanoparticles showed a spontaneous erection (within 5 min of administering the topical agent) and lasted a very short time (1.42 min). Sialorphin nanoparticles also showed spontaneous erections (within 5 min of administering the topical agent) but lasted a longer duration (8 min).

Tadalafil nanoparticles also increased erectile function, but a stimulation of the cavernous nerve was needed to elicit a response. The erectile response was significantly greater approximately 1 h after treatment. Although an increased erectile function was seen with the three different nanoparticles, the time of onset and amount of response was different among the three nanoparticles used. These differences may be due to several factors: molecule size, hydrophobicity, biochemical mechanisms of action and other characteristics of the nanoparticles that may affect the efficiency of transdermal transport, pharmacokinetics and release the erectogenic agents in corporal tissue. Even though no human trials exist yet, the results of this study are promising. Nanoparticles could become a potential new route for topical delivery of a known class of drugs for erectile dysfunction such as PDE5 inhibitors. The added benefits of local therapy resides in avoiding first-pass metabolism, avoiding variations in absorption profiles caused by different foods (high fat food, grapefruit) [67, 68], as well as decreasing systemic side effects (headache, facial flushing, nasal congestion, and dyspepsia).

Furthermore, the previous study showed nanoparticles as a potential delivery system for new erectogenic agents such as NO and sialorphin. As mentioned earlier, in the past, direct application of NO has not been feasible. It is through improvements in the gel structure of nanoparticles that allowed sustained release NO-releasing nanoparticles become possible. Furthermore, NO release could be tuned through manipulation of the components comprising the particles.

Sialorphin has been demonstrated to improve erectile function via intracorporeal injection in animal models. Should its application be translated into clinical treatment in humans, it would involve intracorporeal injection as well. However, topical application via nanoparticles would be easier, less invasive, and more "patient friendly".

Based on their flexibility in carrying different therapeutic agents and their simple use, nanoparticles are promising in the treatment of erectile dysfunction. Further studies are needed to establish their safety in human clinical trials.

Low Intensity Extracorporeal Shock Wave Therapy

Low-intensity extracorporeal shock wave therapy (LI-ESWT) is a recently reported treatment modality for erectile dysfunction. It is well tolerated, noninvasive, and completely safe with no adverse effects reported. Unlike the most commonly used "on demand" and temporary treatments that don't address the pathophysiology of erectile dysfunction (ED), LI-ESWT is rehabilitative and restorative of the underlying mechanism of erectile function with documented long-term improvements.

Shock Waves (SW) are acoustic waves that carry energy which, depending on their intensity level, have various therapeutic applications. High intensity shock waves have mechanical destructive properties; they are used for lithotripsy in the management of kidney stones.

Medium-intensity shock waves have anti-inflammatory properties; they are used to treat different inflammatory conditions. Low intensity shock waves have angiogenic properties; therefore, they are used for their neovascularization effects on chronic wounds, peripheral neuropathy, and cardiac neovascularization, and more recently, as a potential treatment for erectile dysfunction. It is believed that the microtrauma created by focused LI-ESWT on tissue cause the release of angiogenic factors that result in neovascularization. In the 1990s, Young and Dyson first described the effect of ultrasound on tissue angiogenesis [69]. Since then, different animal studies showed that LI-ESWT increases vascular endothelial growth factor (VEGF) among other angiogenesis-related growth factors [70–74]. Furthermore, LI-ESWT was found to enhance the recruitment of stem cells, which themselves contribute to neovascularization of ischemic tissue [75].

The first clinical study on LI-ESWT effect on erectile dysfunction was conducted by Vardi and colleagues in 2010 [76]. Twenty patients with mild to moderate erectile dysfunction were enrolled in the study, and 15 out of those 20 patients showed a significant improvement following LI-ESWT, with an average increase of 7.4 points in the International Index of Erectile Function—Erectile Function (IIEF-EF) domain score. Improved results were reported at 1 month and remained unchanged at 6 months. Using the same treatment protocol and study parameters, the same group conducted a randomized, double-blind, controlled study in 2012 investigating the effects of LI-ESWT on erectile function and penile blood flow on 60 men with erectile dysfunction [77].

Similarly to the previous study, a significant improvement in erectile function was found in the treated group, as compared to the control (sham) group. An objective improvement in erectile function was documented by an in improvement in cavernosal blood flow, as measured by venous occlusion plethysmography of the penis. The results of this study are significant; however, it is limited with the small number of patients enrolled. Larger randomized controlled studies are needed to validate these results. Also in this study, only patients with erectile dysfunction of vasculogenic origin were enrolled.

A better understanding of erectile dysfunction post radical prostatectomy showed that it is more complex than a merely cavernous nerve injury, and that arteriogenic [78–80] and venogenic [9, 81, 82] factors contribute to its pathophysiology. Therefore, LI-ESWT with its neovascularization effect might improve erectile function recovery after the surgery. In this aspect, further studies are needed to investigate the effects of LI-ESWT on ED post-radical prostatectomy. Studies to optimize the treatment protocol (dosage, frequency, and duration of treatment) are needed as well.

Impulse Magnetic Field Therapy

Like LI-ESWT, impulse magnetic field therapy has been investigated as a noninvasive treatment for ED. The rationale behind this form of therapy is that magnetic stimulation induces an alternating electric current within the body's electrolytes which results in changing cellular nutrient exchange, cellular membrane permeability, and other morphologic and physiologic changes within the cell. At certain dosage, this can increase cellular oxygenation and improve blood circulation. Small studies were conducted, including one double blinded placebo-controlled study [83, 84], which documented the improvement of erectile function with this form of therapy. Larger studies are required to further investigate its effectiveness and side effects.

Vibrators and External Penile Support Devices

Vibrators use vibratory stimulation of the penile shaft to help induce erection in patients with erectile dysfunction. They are also used to provoke ejaculation in patients who suffer from a spinal cord injury. Viberect® (Reflexonic, LLC Chambersburg, PA, USA) was the first vibrator to be approved by the FDA in 2011. Vibratory stimulation has been shown to induce the release of NO and other neurotransmitters from terminal nerve endings [85]. These neurotransmitters are involved in the physiology of penile erection. Viberect® has been suggested to be used as an option in penile rehabilitation after radical prostatectomy. A prospective randomized trial conducted by Fode and colleagues compared the effect of penile vibratory stimulation (PVS) plus oral PDE5 inhibitors versus oral PDE5 inhibitors alone in penile rehabilitation following radical prostatectomy [86]. The study showed better IIEF scores at 3, 6, and 12 months after surgery in patients who received penile vibratory stimulation. However, the differences between the two groups were not statistically significant. More clinical trials are needed to confirm the benefits of PVS in the management of penile rehabilitation after radical prostatectomy.

External penile support devices are worn during sexual intercourse and provide penile support and rigidity. There have been no studies to document their efficacy, however recent devices with their unique and innovative designs require further exploration [54].

Tissue Engineering

Many attempts were made throughout history to create a biological penile prosthesis. In 1936, bone cartilage was used in the first known biological reconstruction of the phallus. Later, bovine chondrocytes were used to create cartilaginous rods that were implanted into the corporal spaces in animal studies [87, 88]. In 2002, Kershen and colleagues constructed a neocorpora by seeding human corporal smooth muscle cells on polymer scaffolds [89]. In 2010, Chen and colleagues replaced excised pendular penile corpora cavities in rabbits with three-dimensional (3D) corporal collagen matrices seeded with smooth muscle and endothelial cells [90]. They demonstrated that the neocorpora created exhibited physiological functions such as the ability to attain erection, relax under the effect of NO, and allow intravaginal ejaculation. No human studies have been conducted yet. However, with the major advances and precision in three-dimensional bio-printing, the future of tissue engineering is very promising.

Conclusions

The use of dHAM as a nerve wrap over the preserved NVBs during robotic radical prostatectomy has a significant positive impact on early recovery of erectile function. We have been using dHAM as an adjunctive measure in appropriately selected patients undergoing RALP for over 4 years now. With meticulously performed bilateral nerve preservation the use of dHAM has shown immense promise in the early return of erectile function in our hands.

The concept of postprostatectomy penile rehabilitation is well established now. Early treatment to achieve erection may improve long-term erectile function recovery of spontaneous erections or response to treatment by minimizing penile structural changes. Until now, there has not been any standardized regimen or specific recommendations or guidelines for an optimal penile rehabilitation strategy. Therefore, these therapies are applied differently in various clinical practice patterns, according to physicians' and patients' preferences. At our International Robotic Prostatectomy Institute we routinely start our robotic prostatectomy patients on a rigorous penile rehabilitation program with PDE-5 inhibitors and a vacuum erection device (VED) on the first postoperative visit for catheter removal.

References

1. Dubbelman D, Dohle R, Schroder H. Sexual function before and after radical retropubic prostatectomy: a systemic review of prognostic indicators for successful outcome. Eur Urol. 2006;50:711–8.
2. Mulhall J. Defining and reporting erectile function outcomes after radical prostatectomy: challenges and miscoceptions. J Urol. 2009;181:462–71.
3. Dahm P, Stoffs T, Canfield SE. Recovery of erectile function after robotic prostatectomy: evidence based outcomes. Urol Clin N Am. 2011;38(24):6.
4. Fairbain NG, Redmond RW. The clinical application of human amnion in plastic surgery. J Plast Reconstr Aesthet Surg. 2014;67(5):665–75.
5. Fesli A, Yilmaz N, Comelekoglu U, Tasdelen B. Enhancement of nerve healing with the combined use of amniotic membrane and granulocyte colony stimulation factor. J Plast Reconstr Aesthet Surg. 2014;67(5):837–43.

6. Kim N, Verdi Y, Padma-Nathan H, Daley J, Goldstein I, Saenz de Tejada I. Oxygen tension regulates the nitric oxide pathway. Physiologic role in penile erection. J Clin Invest. 1993;91:437–42.
7. Klein L, Miller M, Buttyan R, et al. Apoptosis in the rat penis after penile denervation. J Urol. 1997;158:626–30.
8. Lue T, Tanagho E. Physiology of erection and pharmacological management of impotence. J Urol. 1987;137:829–36.
9. Mulhall J, Slovick R, Hotaling J, et al. Erectile dysfunction after radical prostatectomy: hemodynamic profiles and their correlation with recovery of erectile function. J Urol. 2002;167:1371–5.
10. Montorsi F, Guazzoni G, Strambi LF, et al. Recovery of spontaneous erectile function after nerve-sparing radical retropubic prostatectomy with and without early intracavernous injections of alprostadil: results of a prospective, randomized trial. J Urol. 1997;158:1408–10.
11. Nandipati K, Raina R, Agarwal A, et al. Early combination therapy: intracavernosal injections and sildenafil following radical prostatectomy increases sexual activity and the return of natural erections. Int J Impot Res. 2006;18:446–51.
12. Bannowsky A, Schulze H, van der Horst C, et al. Recovery of erectile function after nerve-sparing radical prostatectomy: improvement with nightly low-dose sildenafil. BJU Int. 2008;101:1279–83.
13. Mulhall J, Land S, Parker M, et al. The use of an erectogenic pharmacotherapy regimen following radical prostatectomy improves recovery of spontaneous erectile function. J Sex Med. 2005;2:532–40. discussion 540–2.
14. Padma-Nathan H, McCullough AR, Levine LA, Lipshultz LI, Siegel R, et al. Randomized, double-blind, placebo-controlled study of postoperative nightly sildenafil citrate for the prevention of erectile dysfunction after bilateral nerve-sparing radical prostatectomy. Int J Impot Res. 2008;20:479–86.
15. Mulhall JP, Burnett AL, Wang R, McVary KT, Moul JW, et al. A phase 3, placebo controlled study of the safety and efficacy of avanafil for the treatment of erectile dysfunction after nerve sparing radical prostatectomy. J Urol. 2013;189:2229–36.
16. Teloken P, Mesquita G, Montorsi F, Mulhall J. Post-radical prostatectomy pharmacological penile rehabilitation: practice patterns among the international society for sexual medicine practitioners. J Sex Med. 2009;6(7):2032–8.
17. Mulhall JP, Bella AJ, Briganti A, McCullough A, Brock G. Erectile function rehabilitation in the radical prostatectomy patient. J Sex Med. 2010;7(4 Pt 2):1687–98.
18. Schwartz EJ, Wong P, Graydon RJ. Sildenafil preserves intracorporeal smooth muscle after radical retropubic prostatectomy. J Urol. 2004;171(2 Pt 1):771–4.
19. Köhler TS, Pedro R, Hendlin K, Utz W, Ugarte R, Reddy P, et al. A pilot study on the early use of the vacuum erection device after radical retropubic prostatectomy. BJU Int. 2007;100(4):858–62.
20. Raina R, Agarwal A, Ausmundson S, Lakin M, Nandipati KC, Montague DK, et al. Early use of vacuum constriction device following radical prostatectomy facilitates early sexual activity and potentially earlier return of erectile function. Int J Impot Res. 2006;18(1):77–81.
21. Chung E, Brock G. Sexual rehabilitation and cancer survivorship: a state of art review of current literature and management strategies in male sexual dysfunction among prostate cancer survivors. J Sex Med. 2013;10 Suppl 1:102–11.
22. Salonia A, Burnett AL, Graefen M, Hatzimouratidis K, Montorsi F, Mulhall JP, et al. Prevention and management of postprostatectomy sexual dysfunctions. Part 1: choosing the right patient at the right time for the right surgery. Eur Urol. 2012;62(2):261–72.
23. Chung E, Brock GB. Emerging and novel therapeutic approaches in the treatment of male erectile dysfunction. Curr Urol Rep. 2011;12(6):432–43.
24. García-Cardoso J, Vela R, Mahillo E, Mateos-Cáceres PJ, Modrego J, Macaya C, et al. Increased cyclic guanosine monophosphate production and endothelial nitric oxide synthase level in mononuclear cells from sildenafil citrate-treated patients with erectile dysfunction. Int J Impot Res. 2010;22(1):68–76.
25. Montorsi F, Brock G, Lee J, Shapiro J, Van Poppel H, et al. Effect of nightly versus on-demand vardenafil on recovery of erectile function in men following bilateral nerve-sparing radical prostatectomy. Eur Urol. 2008;54:924–31.

26. Montorsi F, Brock G, Stolzenburg JU, Mulhall J, Moncada I, et al. Effects of tadalafil treatment on erectile function recovery following bilateral nerve-sparing radical prostatectomy: a randomised placebo-controlled study (REACTT). Eur Urol. 2014;65:587–96.
27. Natali A, Masieri L, Lanciotti M, Giancane S, Vignolini G, Carini M, et al. A comparison of different oral therapies versus no treatment for erectile dysfunction in 196 radical nerve-sparing radical prostatectomy patients. Int J Impot Res. 2015;27(1):1–5.
28. Segal R, Burnett AL. Avanafil for the treatment of erectile dysfunction. Drugs Today. 2012;48(1):7–15.
29. Paick JS, Kim JJ, Kim SC, et al. Efficacy and safety of mirodenafil in men taking antihypertensive medications. J Sex Med. 2010;7(9):3143–52.
30. Toque HA, Teixeira CE, Lorenzetti R, Okuyama CE, Antunes E, De Nucci G. Pharmacological characterization of a novel phosphodiesterase type 5 (PDE5) inhibitor lodenafil carbonate on human and rabbit corpus cavernosum. Eur J Pharmacol. 2008;591(1–3):189–95.
31. Alba F, Wang R. Current status of penile rehabilitation after radical prostatectomy. J Urol. 2010;16:93–101.
32. McCullough AR, Hellstrom WG, Wang R, Lepor H, Wagner KR, Engel JD. Recovery of erectile function after nerve sparing radical prostatectomy and penile rehabilitation with nightly intraurethral alprostadil versus sildenafil citrate. J Urol. 2010;183:2451–6.
33. Albersen M, Shindel AW, Lue TF. Sexual dysfunction in the older man. Rev Clin Gerontol. 2009;19(4):237–48.
34. Raina R, Pahlajani G, Agarwal A, Zippe CD. The early use of transurethral alprostadil after radical prostatectomy potentially facilitates an earlier return of erectile function and successful sexual activity. BJU Int. 2007;100(6):1317–21.
35. Burnett AL. Erectile dysfunction following radical prostatectomy. JAMA. 2005;293:2648–53.
36. Claro JA, de Aboim JE, Maríngolo M, Andrade E, Aguiar W, Nogueira M, et al. Intracavernous injection in the treatment of erectile dysfunction after radical prostatectomy: an observational study. Sao Paulo Med J. 2001;119:135–7.
37. Gontero P, Fontana F, Bagnasacco A, Panella M, Kocjancic E, Pretti G, et al. Is there an optimal time for intracavernous prostaglandin E1 rehabilitation following nonnerve sparing radical prostatectomy? Results from a hemodynamic prospective study. J Urol. 2003;169(6):2166–9.
38. Mulhall JP, Parker M, Waters BW, Flanigan R. The timing of penile rehabilitation after bilateral nerve-sparing radical prostatectomy affects the recovery of erectile function. BJU Int. 2010;105:37–41.
39. Yiou R, Tow BZ, Parisot J, et al. Is it worth continuing sexual rehabilitation after radical prostatectomy with intracavernous injection of alprostadil for more than 1 year? J Sex Med. 2015;3:42–8.
40. Lewis R, Witherington R. External vacuum therapy for erectile dysfunction: use and results. World J Urol. 1997;15:78–82.
41. Brison D, Seftel A, Sadeghi-Nejad H. The resurgence of the vacuum erection device (VED) for treatment of erectile dysfunction. J Sex Med. 2013;10:1124–35.
42. Lin H, Yang W, Zhang J, Dai Y, Wang R. Penile rehabilitation with a vacuum erectile device in an animal model is related to an antihypoxic mechanism: blood gas evidence. Asian J Androl. 2013;15:387–90.
43. Yuan J, Hoang A, Romero C, Lin H, Dai Y, Wang R. Vacuum therapy in erectile dysfunction — science and clinical evidence. Int J Impot Res. 2010;22:211–9.
44. Yuan J, Lin H, Li P, Zhang R, Luo A, Berardinelli F, et al. Molecular mechanisms of vacuum therapy in penile rehabilitation: a novel animal study. Eur Urol. 2010;58:773–80.
45. Yuan J, Westney O, Wang R. Design and application of a new rat-specific vacuum erectile device for penile rehabilitation research. J Sex Med. 2009;6:3247–53.
46. Monga M, Utz W, Reddy P, Kohler T, Hendlin K, et al. Early use of the vacuum constriction device following radical retropubic prostatectomy: a randomized clinical trial south central section of the AUA 85th annual meeting; 2006. p. 98.
47. Bosshardt RJ, Farwerk R, Sikora R, Sohn M, Jakse G. Objective measurement of the effectiveness, therapeutic success and dynamic mechanisms of the vacuum device. Br J Urol. 1995;75:786–91.

48. Gontero P, Fontana F, Zitella A, Montorsi F, Frea B. A prospective evaluation of efficacy and compliance with a multistep treatment approach for erectile dysfunction in patients after non-nerve sparing radical prostatectomy. BJU Int. 2005;95:359–65.
49. Raina R, Agarwal A, Allamaneni SS, Lakin MM, Zippe CD. Sildenafil citrate and vacuum constriction device combination enhances sexual satisfaction in erectile dysfunction after radical prostatectomy. Urology. 2005;65:360–4.
50. Raina R, Pahlajani G, Agarwal A, Jones S, Zippe C. Long-term potency after early use of a vacuum erection device following radical prostatectomy. BJU Int. 2010;106:1719–22.
51. Engel JD. Effect on sexual function of a vacuum erection device post-prostatectomy. Can J Urol. 2011;18:5721–5.
52. Basal S, Wambi C, Acikel C, Gupta M, Badani K. Optimal strategy for penile rehabilitation after robot-assisted radical prostatectomy based on preoperative erectile function. BJU Int. 2013;111:658–65.
53. Montorsi F, Adaikan G, Becher E, et al. Summary of the recommendations on sexual dysfunctions in men. J Sex Med. 2010;7(11):3572–88.
54. Stein M, Lin H. New advances in erectile technology. Ther Adv Urol. 2014;6(1):15–24.
55. Lim P. Recent advances and research updates. 2003. ISSN-0972-4689.
56. Le B, Colombo A, Mustoe T, McVary K. Evaluation of a Ni-Ti shape memory alloy for use in a novel penile prosthesis. J Urol. 2013;189(Suppl):502.
57. Swords K, Martinez D, Lockhart J, Carrion R. A preliminary report on the usage of an intracorporeal antibiotic cast with synthetic high purity CaSO4 for the treatment of infected penile implant. J Sex Med. 2013;10:1162–9.
58. Yap RL, Mcvary KT. Topical agents and erectile dysfunction: is there a place? Curr Urol Rep. 2002;3:471–6.
59. Montorsi F, Salonia A, Zanoni M, Pompa P, Cestari A, Guazzoni G, et al. Current status of local penile therapy. Int J Impot Res. 2002;14(1 suppl):S70–81.
60. Friedman AJ, Han G, Navati MS, Chacko M, Gunther L, Alfieri A, et al. Sustained release nitric oxide releasing nanoparticles: characterization of a novel delivery platform based on nitrite containing hydrogel/glass composites. Nitric Oxide. 2008;19:12–20.
61. Gupta R, Kumar A. Bioactive materials for biomedical applications using sol-gel technology. Biomed Mater. 2008;3:034005.
62. Khan I, Dantsker D, Samuni U, Friedman AJ, Bonaventura C, Manjula B, et al. Beta 93 modified hemoglobin: kinetic and conformational consequences. Biochemistry. 2001;40:7581–92.
63. Khan I, Shannon CF, Dantsker D, Friedman AJ, Perez-Gonzalez-de-Apodaca J, Friedman JM. Sol-gel trapping of functional intermediates of hemoglobin: geminate and bimolecular recombination studies. Biochemistry. 2000;39:16099–109.
64. Viitala R, Jokinen M, Rosenholm JB. Mechanistic studies on release of large and small molecules from biodegradable SiO2. Int J Pharm. 2007;336:382–90.
65. Han G, Tar M, Kuppam D, Friedman A, Melman A, Friedman J, et al. Nanoparticles as a novel delivery vehicle for therapeutics targeting erectile dysfunction. J Sex Med. 2010;7:224–33.
66. Davies KP, Tar M, Rougeot C, Melman A. Sialorphin (the mature peptide product of Vcsa1) relaxes corporal smooth muscle tissue and increases erectile function in the ageing rat. BJU Int. 2007;99:431–5.
67. Seftel AD. Phosphodiesterase type 5 inhibitor differentiation based on selectivity, pharmacokinetic, and efficacy profiles. Clin Cardiol. 2004;27(4 suppl 1):114–9.
68. Jetter A, Kinzig-Schippers M, Walchner-Bonjean M, Hering U, Bulitta J, Schreiner P, et al. Effects of grapefruit juice on the pharmacokinetics of sildenafil. Clin Pharmacol Ther. 2002;71:21–9.
69. Young S, Dyson M. The effect of therapeutic ultrasound on angiogenesis. Ultrasound Med Biol. 1990;16:261–9.
70. Qiu X, Lin G, Xin Z, Ferretti L, Zhang H, Lue T, et al. Effects of low-energy shockwave therapy on the erectile function and tissue of a diabetic rat model. J Sex Med. 2013;10:738–46.
71. Wang C, Huang H, Pai C. Shock wave-enhanced neovascularization at the tendon-bone junction: an experiment in dogs. J Foot Ankle Surg. 2002;41:16–22.

72. Wang C, Wang F, Yang K, Weng L, Hsu C, Huang C, et al. Shock wave therapy induces neo-vascularization at the tendon-bone junction. A study in rabbits. J Orthop Res. 2003;21:984–9.
73. Gutersohn A, Caspari G, Vopahl M, Erbel R. Upregulation of VEGF mRNA in HUVEC via shock waves. In: Proceedings of the international conference from genes to therapy in ischemic and heart muscle disease, Marburg, Germany, 9–10 Oct 1999.
74. Nishida T, Shimokawa H, Oi K, Tatewaki H, Uwatoku T, Abe T, et al. Extracorporeal cardiac shock wave therapy markedly ameliorates ischemia-induced myocardial dysfunction in pigs in vivo. Circulation. 2004;110:3055–61.
75. Aicher A, Heeschen C, Sasaki K, Urbich C, Zeiher A, Dimmeler S. Low-energy shock wave for enhancing recruitment of endothelial progenitor cells: a new modality to increase efficacy of cell therapy in chronic hind limb ischemia. Circulation. 2006;114:2823–30.
76. Vardi Y, Appel B, Jacob G, Massarwi O, Gruenwald I. Can low-intensity extracorporeal shock-wave therapy improve erectile function? A 6-month follow-up pilot study in patients with organic erectile dysfunction. Eur Urol. 2010;58:243–8.
77. Vardi Y, Appel B, Kilchevsky A, Gruenwald I. Does low intensity extracorporeal shock wave therapy have a physiological effect on erectile function? Short-term results of a randomized, double-blind, sham controlled study. J Urol. 2012;187:1769–75.
78. Walz J, Burnett AL, Costello AJ, Eastham JA, Graefen M, Guillonneau B, et al. A critical analysis of the current knowledge of surgical anatomy related to optimization of cancer control and preservation of continence and erection in candidates for radical prostatectomy. Eur Urol. 2010;57:179–92.
79. Rogers CG, Trock BP, Walsh PC. Preservation of accessory pudendal arteries during radical retropubic prostatectomy: surgical technique and results. Urology. 2004;64:148–51.
80. Mulhall JP, Secin FP, Guillonneau B. Artery sparing radical prostatectomy – myth or reality? J Urol. 2008;179:827–31.
81. Moreland RB. Is there a role of hypoxemia in penile fibrosis: a viewpoint presented to the Society for the Study of Impotence. Int J Impot Res. 1998;10:113–20.
82. Nehra A, Hall SJ, Basile G, Bertero EB, Moreland R, Toselli P, et al. Systemic sclerosis and impotence: a clinicopathological correlation. J Urol. 1995;153:1140–6.
83. Pelka R, Jaenicke C, Gruenwald J. Impulse magnetic-field therapy for erectile dysfunction: a double-blind, placebo-controlled study. Adv Ther. 2002;19:53–60.
84. Shafik A, El-Sibai O, Shafik A. Magnetic stimulation of the cavernous nerve for the treatment of erectile dysfunction in humans. Int J Impot Res. 2000;12:137–41. discussion 141–132.
85. Tajkarimi K, Burnett A. Viberect® device use by men with erectile dysfunction: safety, ease of use, tolerability, and satisfaction survey. J Sex Med. 2011;8:441.
86. Fode M, Borre M, Ohl DA, Lichtbach J, Sønksen J. Penile vibratory stimulation in the recovery of urinary continence and erectile function after nerve-sparing radical prostatectomy: a randomized, controlled trial. BJU Int. 2014;114:111–7.
87. Yoo J, Lee I, Atala A. Cartilage rods as a potential material for penile reconstruction. J Urol. 1998;160:1164–8. discussion 1178.
88. Yoo J, Park H, Lee I, Atala A. Autologous engineered cartilage rods for penile reconstruction. J Urol. 1999;162:1119–21.
89. Kershen R, Yoo J, Moreland R, Krane R, Atala A. Reconstitution of human corpus cavernosum smooth muscle in vitro and in vivo. Tissue Eng. 2002;8:515–24.
90. Chen K, Eberli D, Yoo J, Atala A. Bioengineered corporal tissue for structural and functional restoration of the penis. Proc Natl Acad Sci U S A. 2010;107:3346–50.

Index

© Springer International Publishing Switzerland 2016
S. Razdan (ed.), *Urinary Continence and Sexual Function After Robotic Radical Prostatectomy*, DOI 10.1007/978-3-319-39448-0